THE HORRORS OF HOLISTIC MEDICINE

June B. Schmidt

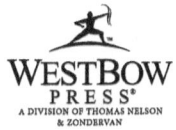

WESTBOW
PRESS®
A DIVISION OF THOMAS NELSON
& ZONDERVAN

Scripture quotations are from the Revised Standard Version of the Bible,
copyright © 1946, 1952, and 1971 National Council of the Churches of Christ
in the United States of America. Used by permission. All rights reserved.

WestBow Press books may be ordered through booksellers or by contacting:

WestBow Press
A Division of Thomas Nelson & Zondervan
1663 Liberty Drive
Bloomington, IN 47403
www.westbowpress.com
1 (866) 928-1240

ISBN: 978-1-5127-6927-2 (sc)
ISBN: 978-1-5127-6928-9 (hc)
ISBN: 978-1-5127-6926-5 (e)

Library of Congress Control Number: 2016921043

Print information available on the last page.

WestBow Press rev. date: 05/23/2019

CONTENTS

Acknowledgments vii

Chapter 1—"Cancer?" 1

Chapter 2—"I Could Have Died" 6

Chapter 3—"We Treat the 'Whole' Person" 11

Chapter 4—The Holistic Bubble Bursts 22

Chapter 5—"Your Medicine Is Doing You No Good" 33

Chapter 6—"Do You Hate Me?" 40

Chapter 7—"Your Test for Lupus Was Slightly Positive" 45

Chapter 8—"It Could Be Cancer" 53

Chapter 9—"Three Years to Live" 59

Chapter 10—Tests and Questions 66

Chapter 11—The Decision Is Made 72

Chapter 12—Two Friends: the Old 78

Chapter 13—Two Friends: the New 92

Chapter 14—"You Didn't Have the Pain" 103

Chapter 15—Surgery 111

Chapter 16—"They Don't Give Medals for Enduring Pain" 120

Chapter 17—The Fear of Not Knowing 127

Chapter 18—"The Battle Has Only Begun ..." 132

Chapter 19—Spiraling Down into Depression 140

Chapter 20—Out of Control 153

Chapter 21—Cryosurgery 166

Chapter 22—"Something is *Still* Wrong" 171

Chapter 23—Quicksand 177

Chapter 24—Test the Spirits 183

Chapter 25—The Fifty-Thousand-Piece Puzzle.............................. 193

Chapter 26—The Mystery Deepens... 197

Chapter 27—"It Could Be Melanoma" 203

Chapter 28—Healed: Body, Mind, and Spirit 210

Appendix A—My Letter to the Arizona Nursing Association........ 219

Appendix B—My Letter to Dr. Johnson, Neurologist 225

ACKNOWLEDGMENTS

First of all, I want to thank my husband, Bud, who traveled this rocky road of deception and healing with me, and remained constant and supportive throughout the entire ordeal.

Special thanks to Carole Farley, my friend, who after seeing a resurgence in New Age "alternative care" health practices, urged me to finish writing this book to expose the deceit of holistic medicine. Without her encouragement, hugs, and editing suggestions, this book would never have been completed.

Thanks also to Millie Barger, my friend and colleague from my Christian writers' club, a published author in her own right, who edited my early drafts and offered valuable suggestions for improvement.

And thanks to all the members of my Christian writers' club who supported me with invaluable suggestions and encouragement during the thirty plus years I labored to complete this manuscript and to put my thoughts into printed form.

I also want to especially thank my two WestBow Press editors, Alex Stine and Jennifer Morris, for all their technical assistance in getting my manuscript into book format. Without their help, this book would never have been finished.

CHAPTER 1

"CANCER?"

"Cancer?" I shook my head in shock and disbelief, refusing to accept the death sentence I thought my gynecologist was pronouncing.

"You have a large mass on your left ovary," he said gently. "It could be cancer."

The nightmare of months of uncertainty and testing had become a horrible reality.

It was March 24, 1982. Just the day before, Dr. Fields,[1] my hematologist, had said, "I can't make an accurate diagnosis until you've seen a gynecologist."

I had first consulted Dr. Fields on October 30, 1981, because my body had not been responding to the anemia treatment recommended by my holistic medical doctor. Three months ago, while searching for the cause of my long-standing anemia, Dr. Fields had off-handedly suggested, "I'd like you to see a gynecologist. Do you know one?"

I didn't have a gynecologist, but I had replied, "I can ask a friend."

"That will be fine," he had responded.

The request had sounded routine, not urgent, not like one that would help make a quicker diagnosis. It had sounded more precautionary, as part of my total health picture. Only four months earlier, I'd had my yearly pelvic and pap tests at Arcadia Clinic, the holistic medical facility I patronized. The licensed nurse practitioner (LNP), who had always

---

[1] Some names, places, and descriptive material have been changed to protect privacy.

1

performed my exams, had reported that everything was "normal." So I had been in no hurry to incur added and unnecessary expense by repeating the procedure without good reason.

It never occurred to me that my holistic practitioner might not be honest or could be mistaken.

In the meantime, however, I'd talked to a friend who gave me the name of her gynecologist. I figured I would visit him next June, around my birthday, when I normally had my annual pelvic and pap exam.

One of the first questions Dr. Fields asked during the March 23 visit was, "Have you seen a gynecologist yet?"

"No," I admitted. "I thought I would wait until June when I normally have that exam."

That's when he explained he could not complete his diagnosis until I was checked. "There's a good gynecologist in this building," he said. "Do you mind if I make an appointment for you?"

"No," I answered cautiously. "Go ahead." Actually, I preferred to have him make the arrangements. Doctors, I believed, were more aware of who in the medical profession were reliable physicians and who were the "quacks." Friends are often swayed by emotional loyalty to their doctors.

I expected the appointment to be made for the following week or even the following month, depending on how busy the doctor's schedule was.

"You have an appointment with Dr. John Lance tomorrow morning at nine-thirty," Dr. Fields said, coming back into the examining room. "I've discussed your case with him. Can you be there?"

"*Tomorrow* morning?" I repeated, believing I had not heard him correctly. Dr. Fields was a tall man. Now, towering above me, he seemed imposingly huge as he peered over his half-glasses and wordlessly nodded his head. "Yes, I suppose I can be there." I was only slightly unnerved by his haste in setting up the appointment. After all, he had suggested it months before. Apparently, however, the recommendation had not been meant as a simple *request*.

Dr. John Lance, a youthful, handsome doctor, had that "all-American boy" look, more like someone who had just graduated from college than a medical school graduate. He reminded me of the type of person I expected to see running for college student-body president.

"You have an abdominal mass about the size of a tennis ball in your left ovary," he reported when he finished the pelvic exam. "It could be cancer."

"How can that be?" I retorted. "I had a pelvic exam last June. I was told everything was 'normal.' *Do cancers grow that fast?*"

"Sometimes they are hard to detect," he replied, smoothly sidestepping my question.

I raised my voice in frustration. "Well, I've had the pain for at least ten years. Certainly they should have felt *something* in that length of time."

Ignoring my anger, Dr. Lance maneuvered the conversation back to the issue at hand. "You have a large abdominal mass. It needs to come out as soon as possible. You also have some large fibroids in the uterus, and there probably is endometriosis."

"No one ever told me I had fibroids, but I know I have endometriosis. I've had it for years. Betty said it was nothing to worry about; that it would go away when I finished menopause; that it would dry up with my periods." Betty, the middle-aged grandmotherly nurse practitioner who performed my gynecological exams at the holistic clinic which I'd patronized for the last sixteen years, never had given me any reason to think I might have a problem. Every year she announced, "Everything is normal."

"In cases like this," Dr. Lance continued, "we recommend an immediate complete hysterectomy—removal of both ovaries, fallopian tubes, uterus, everything. At your age, it doesn't pay to leave something and have to go back in a few years to remove something else."

I was forty-three years old, childless, and never considered myself a candidate for hysterectomy. Instead, my husband, Bud, and I hoped for a premenopausal baby.

As I look back now, I realize how outlandish my excuses to the doctor must have sounded.

"I can't have surgery now," I argued, "My oldest niece is getting married in Minnesota in July. We're flying back for the wedding. And I edit a newsletter for our district women's group. Our executive board meets in California next month. I have to be there. And at the end of May, my husband's parents are celebrating their fiftieth wedding anniversary. We're hosting the open house at our place." One excuse begot another. I shook my head, determined to delay the surgery. "It takes too long to recover from a hysterectomy—weeks, even months. I don't want to miss any of those events. Maybe in August"—I mentally scanned my schedule—"when all those activities are over. Maybe then we can talk about scheduling surgery."

"If it's cancer, you don't want to wait," Dr. Lance emphasized.

It was a simple, direct statement of fact. The seriousness of the situation quickly put everything into proper perspective. Cancer. The ominous word struck me like a bullet. Cancer of the female organs.

Since I'd first seen Dr. Fields in October 1981 for unresolved anemia, cancer had lurked in the back of my mind. But based on a variety of symptoms, the cancers I had considered were leukemia, lymphoma, bone cancer, or lung cancer. Why hadn't I ever considered cancer of the ovaries? That's where all the pain had been—for ten years or more.

In 1965, when I became a patient at Arcadia Clinic, holistic medicine was a new concept in health care. They claimed to treat the "whole person"—body, mind, and spirit. As a Christian, the concept of whole-person health care appealed to me. I did all the things they advised. I practiced preventive medicine. I followed good nutrition. I didn't drink hard liquor or smoke. I took care of my body as they said I should. *How could I have cancer?*

In 1973, Dr. Jim Barry, my holistic doctor, said I was anemic. Since then, iron preparations, both in tablet form and shots, and an assortment of vitamins in large doses were the recommended treatments by my holistic healers. None of the doctors or Betty, the LNP, ever resolved the anemia, which they nonchalantly referred to as a "stubborn case."

When I finally consulted Dr. Fields, I complained of overwhelming fatigue. Tiredness dogged my days and had for many years. I made excuses to myself for the fatigue: I was too busy and didn't give myself enough time for relaxation. But even sitting still, I could not relax. I was restless; I needed to be doing something *all the time*, but I never seemed to get much accomplished. If I had been a child, I probably would have been diagnosed as hyperactive. I couldn't seem to get organized, to set goals, or to complete projects. I felt like a car spinning its wheels in fresh snow or deep sand. Although I expended a lot of energy, I wasn't going anywhere or making forward progress. Now, I began to wonder if my "too active" lifestyle was the real cause for the fatigue.

My right hand brushed the air, a gesture of both futility and despair, as I tried to sweep away the words that hung like cobwebs in front of my face. The reality of cancer—serious, chronic illness—seeped slowly into my conscious mind and wormed its way down into the depths of my soul.

"Yes," I finally and fearfully acknowledged to Dr. Lance as resignation crept into my voice. "Yes, I suppose cancer would explain the anemia, wouldn't it? I suppose that's why Dr. Fields made this appointment so quickly."

Later that evening, at home, as I reflected on the events of the last sixteen years as a patient at Arcadia Clinic, I wondered, *How did I get myself into this situation?*

I had completed college. I'd worked as an advertising copywriter with a large company for many years. How could I have been so easily and completely fooled by my medical providers?

CHAPTER 2

"I COULD HAVE DIED"

Prior to joining the Arcadia Clinic, I had a frightening experience with another medical doctor.

In 1964, I experienced a loss of feeling in my left foot and leg below the knee. I visited Dr. Ben Spence, a metabolic specialist, whose office was in my neighborhood. The numbness came on quickly, over a weekend, which justifiably alarmed me.

After administering a five-hour glucose tolerance test, Dr. Spence diagnosed me with sugar diabetes. Although my glucose (blood sugar) count of two hundred might have suggested treatment with diet alone, Dr. Spence recommended an oral anti-diabetic prescription tablet, Dymelor. Perhaps he felt the need for more drastic, immediate treatment because of the numbness in my leg. When writing the prescription, Dr. Spence stressed two points: (1) "Take your medicine on time," and (2) "Don't skip any meals or doses." The tablets were to be taken twice a day, twelve hours apart. He gave me no cautionary information, nor did he even suggest the possibility of a hypoglycemic (low blood sugar) reaction.

Two days later, a Saturday, I experienced shakiness. All my nerves felt on edge. I called Dr. Spence at his office (fortunately, he had Saturday morning office hours) and reported my symptoms. Although I had already displayed the classic symptoms of hypoglycemia, his simplistic suggestion was "Eat more." He did not request to see me. He did not suggest that I discontinue taking the Dymelor. He did not tell me to add something sweet to my diet to counterbalance the low blood sugar. Nor did he even suggest that I might be experiencing a *low blood sugar reaction*.

The next day I experienced all the helplessness and horror of a severe hypoglycemic reaction, not once but twice in the same day. Because I had been cautioned not to miss a single dose, I continued to take my medicine when I should not have taken any.

Saturday night's pill was taken at eight o'clock. Overnight, my blood sugar dropped so low that I failed to wake up the next morning at my usual seven o'clock wake-up time. When I did wake and looked at the clock, it was 10:00 a.m. All I could think was, *I'm late for my Sunday school class*—I taught sixth grade. I jumped out of bed, in a hurry to get dressed, and my legs crumbled beneath me like jelly. I fell to the floor, and my face hit the tile floor with such force that I chipped a large piece from one front tooth (although I didn't realize this until several hours later when I looked in a mirror). My body felt numb all over. I was unmarried and living alone. I knew I needed help, so I crawled to my front door, fumbling with the doorknob. The numbness in my fingers prevented me from getting a firm grip on the doorknob. Turning it seemed impossible. I prayed, "God help me."

Finally, it opened. I just yelled, "Help!" My landlady, working outside, heard my cries. "I'm diabetic," I said.

She knew what to do. She gave me a glass of orange juice, which soon revived me and in a short time restored feeling to my body. Shakily, I stood up, but remembering my doctor's admonition not to skip a single dose, I took the 8:00 a.m. pill. It was close to noon.

No one had warned me that when this type of reaction occurs, I should stop taking all medication and call my doctor or go to the nearest hospital emergency department immediately.

Friends had invited me to dinner that day. I called them to cancel, explaining what had happened. Fortunately, they refused to let me cancel. "We'll be right down to get you," Johnnie said.

Johnnie was an artist in the advertising and public relations department for the company where I worked as an advertising copywriter. He and his wife, Dorothy, were an older, childless couple and had befriended me since I had no family in Arizona, and neither did they. That Sunday they took me to their house to spend the day.

Unable to reach Dr. Spence on Sunday, we stopped at the nearest hospital's emergency department on our way to their house. After hearing my story, the ER doctor warned of a possible *second reaction* and ordered, "*Stop* taking that medication."

I spent the rest of the day with Dorothy and Johnnie, waiting for the second reaction to occur. They plied me with orange juice and food. Although I wasn't hungry, I ate because I knew it would help. I didn't feel like a very good guest that day because I only wanted to sleep. I slept in their guest bedroom most of the afternoon. After supper, I felt better and more alert. As we visited, the second reaction occurred. It was sudden and unexpected.

I stared at Johnnie. "I can see three of you," I said, and then my speech became garbled. Although my mental processes were intact, I couldn't communicate. Once again numbness spread over my body. The speed with which this happened scared me. I tried desperately to tell them what I was experiencing, but I could not.

Johnnie called Mercy General Hospital and then helped me into their car, and we raced to the emergency entrance. A medical crew awaited us. They quickly drew blood. Then they gave me a shot of glucose directly into the vein. The glucose brought me out of the reaction but left me sleepy and exhausted. About midnight we returned to their house. I stayed overnight. They didn't want to risk my having another reaction with no one to help. In the morning, however, I was fine.

Sometime later, I learned my blood sugar reading was forty when I was brought to the hospital. Thirty-five, I later heard, could be fatal. I thanked God for saving my life.

Although furious with Dr. Spence after the double reaction, I returned to his office. Now he suggested I try controlling my diabetes with diet alone. The helplessness of the hypoglycemic experience so frightened me that I decided if a strict diet could prevent a recurrence, I would choose the diet. I *never* wanted to experience another hypoglycemic reaction.

I learned to plan meals around the seven basic food exchange groups and to eat meals—breakfast, lunch, and supper— at regular intervals. My landlady loaned me her copy of the Joslin Diabetes Center's manual for diabetics.[2] This manual helped me to understand diabetes and how to treat it. The diet was not nearly as restrictive as I expected. Growing up, our family didn't have lots of sweets in the house so I hadn't developed a "sweet tooth." The Joslin Center's good, healthy diet already had me on the road to stabilized diabetic health, but I didn't realize it at the time.

I thought the initial high-glucose reading of two hundred might have caused impaired circulation and thus the numbness in my lower leg. In place of a coffee break, I'd been having a daily afternoon "candy bar" break, which I now discontinued.

But I had lost confidence in Dr. Spence's ability to manage my health care. I was piqued that he had not apologized for making me go through the reaction, especially since I had called him the day *before*, describing all the symptoms of a reaction, and he had not recognized it as a reaction to the medicine. Instead, he excused himself by saying, "You would not have understood a hypoglycemic reaction until you had experienced one"—as if it was my fault.

I retorted, "If you cannot explain a hypoglycemic reaction to me in terms I could understand, you have no business being a doctor. *I could have died.*"

He sat silent. No apology. No excuses.

---

[2] The Joslin Diabetes Center was founded in 1898 in Boston, Massachusetts, and has become the world's foremost institution for diabetes research, clinical care and education. In 1976, they perfected the A1C test to detect for diabetes. Their recent manual is *The Joslin Guide to Diabetes, A Manual for Managing Your Treatment* © 2005. Also, *What You Need to Know About Diabetes - Revised.*

I had picked Dr. Spence's name from the Yellow Pages of the telephone book because his office was in my neighborhood, and I could walk there. I would not make the same mistake again. I called the County Medical Association, asking for their physicians' referral number. Then I requested the name of a good general physician in my area (I had since moved, bought a car, and wanted a doctor closer to my new address). They gave me the name and address of Dr. Jim Berry. Dr. Berry, they said, had recent success treating patients with diabetes.

I looked forward to meeting him, hopeful that my diabetes could be controlled, and I could get on with my life.

CHAPTER 3

"WE TREAT THE 'WHOLE' PERSON"

In the fall of 1965, Dr. Jim had scheduled me for a seven-hour glucose tolerance test. When he got the results, he announced, "You are not diabetic [high blood sugar] after all but hypoglycemic [low blood sugar]." Hypoglycemia, a relatively new diagnosis in the mid-'60s, was considered a pre-diabetic condition. "The standard diet and treatment for both hypoglycemia and diabetes is the same," he counseled. "It's a well-balanced, high-protein nutritional diet that avoids excess sugars and carbohydrates."

This new diagnosis helped me to understand why Dymelor had caused the severe reaction. After six hours without food, my blood sugar fell to abnormally low levels. The medication caused it to continue dropping—*to dangerously low levels*. That I woke up Sunday morning at all was a miracle.

With my health problems now correctly diagnosed and being treated, I began to feel better. Dr. Jim also recommended I take a tablet of "natural organic compounds," which was sold in the clinic's pharmacy, to increase pancreatic activity and, hopefully, restore insulin production to normal. Diabetes, I learned, is caused by the body's inability to release insulin properly. Insulin production is regulated by the pancreatic gland. That hooked me. The pancreatic pill he prescribed for me seemed like magic.

As I regained good health and the feeling of well-being, Dr. Jim and I entered into a friendly doctor/patient trust relationship. Dr. Jim, with his prematurely white hair, reminded me of a benevolent, gentle, grandfatherly person. He seemed almost Godlike in appearance and demeanor, generously sharing his time to listen to my every complaint. This came at a time when doctors were receiving criticism for rushing patients through their appointments in an assembly-line fashion.

Dr. Jim was in practice with his wife, Dr. Mary Berry. Both were members of the American Holistic Medical Association, which professed to treat the whole person—body, mind, and spirit—acknowledging that humans are emotional *and* spiritual beings, as well as physical beings. "The total person contributes to a person's medical makeup and well-being," Dr. Jim explained. As a Christian, I too believed we are more than just physical bodies, that emotional and spiritual disharmony can contribute to illness. From the very beginning, their philosophy of whole-person care attracted me.

The clinic also offered evening Bible studies in their quest to treat the whole person, and they encouraged me to attend. I already was taking instruction in the Bethel Bible series through my church, so I declined this offer. (Later I was glad that I had not gotten involved with their Bible studies, which I now believe fostered spiritual deception and mind control.)

Dr. Jim further clarified that their clinic practiced "preventive medicine"; a healthy body could be achieved and maintained through proper nutrition, exercise, and mental attitude (right thinking). The basic premise was to keep the body's chemistry in proper balance while ridding it of excessive, harmful poisons and toxins that caused disease and illness. They advocated minimal use of "dangerous prescription drugs," preferring to treat the body with non-dangerous vitamins and natural remedies whenever possible. "Natural foods and herbs," Dr. Jim declared, "will not produce toxic buildups or the various side effects often associated with many prescription drugs. Our clinic subscribes to the many teachings of Edgar Cayce, who advocated natural medical remedies to help the body heal itself."

I had never heard of Edgar Cayce, nor did I care what he believed, as long as it worked. Because Dr. Jim had been recommended to me by a reliable resource, the Arizona Medical Association, I expected him to diagnose and treat my health needs according to accepted medical standards. After my close encounter with death from an ill-prescribed prescription drug, I was very attracted to this medical philosophy. "Prescription drugs," Dr. Jim stated, "are prescribed by the clinic *only* as a last resort, if nothing else works." If I could rule my health by diet and exercise and never have to take another prescription pill again, I wanted to try. (How easily we delude ourselves.)

Arcadia Clinic's holistic approach to medicine caused them to grow and thrive. It attracted many people, who recommended the clinic to their friends. When I married in 1967, my husband, Bud, became a patient.

I met Bud at church. He and his parents attended the Bethel Bible class I taught.

For a year after our marriage, because we wanted to make sure our relationship was stable before we started a family, I took birth control pills prescribed by Dr. Jim. Soon after starting that prescription drug, nagging pain troubled me in the lower left quadrant of my abdomen; it was diagnosed as "normal menstrual pain." Menstrual cramps hadn't bothered me for years. I vaguely remembered having them when I was young, soon after I started my menses, but I had been cramp-free for almost fifteen years. I believed the birth control pills contributed to my discomfort.

After a year on the pill, severe nausea attacks accompanied the monthly cramping. When a different prescription birth control pill provided no relief, Dr. Jim suggested, "Why don't you discontinue the pill and start a family?"

I was ready now for this step; I stopped taking birth control pills. The nausea ceased, but the monthly cramps persisted.

As I continued to complain about abdominal pain, Dr. Jim advised me to use castor oil packs with a heating pad, a remedy Edgar Cayce recommended to remove poisonous toxins from the body. The toxins supposedly caused the monthly menstrual discomfort. (Dr. Jim referred to it as a woman's "unclean time," as mentioned in the Bible.) Miraculously, each month after hour-long castor oil pack treatments, the pain ceased, and I felt reassured—until the next month. (Only later did I learn that heat alone is an effective treatment for menstrual pain.) Still, the castor oil packs the clinic promoted seemed to offer a "mysterious" healing quality, except I received no *real* healing.

Our desire for children grew, yet pregnancy eluded us. During one appointment, I wondered aloud to Dr. Jim if a cyst or tumor in my left ovary could be causing the pain and preventing pregnancy. Although I knew very little about human anatomy, the pain seemed localized where I imagined the left ovary to be. Dr. Jim assured me that my yearly pelvic exams showed *no abnormalities*.

However, in 1973, he found what he suspected to be a "small water cyst" on the left ovary. He recommended acupuncture, a new Chinese treatment just gaining popularity in the medical profession. Dr. Jim implied acupuncture would "dry up" the cyst. He had recently returned from attending a special training program in China to learn this new technique. Magically, after a treatment, the pain disappeared. (Years later, I learned that acupuncture, while effective as a pain-blocker, has no curative basis for treating ovarian cysts.)

When the pain returned, I did not associate it with the cyst diagnosis. My doctor assured me the water cyst had dried up. "Menstrual pain—a woman's curse," Dr. Jim counseled. "It's something many women just have to learn to live with." Again, castor oil packs became the recommended treatment. At subsequent yearly pelvic and pap exams, he never mentioned the ovarian cyst.

As years passed, we remained childless and sought advice from Dr. Jim to help us conceive. Once, he suggested that Bud and I have our astrological charts cast to determine if we were capable of conceiving a child together. He gave us the name and address of an astrology center.

The suggestion seemed so preposterous and unscientific to me that

I, tactlessly, laughed out loud in his presence. "Our church doesn't believe in astrology," I clarified. (*And neither do Christians,* I thought, but I didn't say that aloud.)

If he felt insulted by my lack of tact, he didn't show it. Instead, he gently chided, "Do not scoff at things you do not understand." He reproved me but never mentioned the subject of astrology again. Still, his reprimand lay in the back of my mind. Had I scoffed at something I didn't fully understand?

"Bud might have a low sperm count," Dr. Jim suggested one day, but instead of ordering a sperm test, he recommended drinking watermelon-seed tea (available through the clinic's pharmacy), another Edgar Cayce remedy to cleanse the system of "impurities" and increase sperm activity. "It only takes one sperm to impregnate," he added, always dangling hope before us.

Although skeptical about the herbal tea treatment, we had reached a point where we were willing to try almost anything. Even if it didn't help, what could it hurt? I bought the tea. Bud drank one cupful, announcing, "It tastes awful." He refused anymore tea potions.

During one office visit, I asked Dr. Jim if I should see a gynecologist. He took my suggestion as a personal affront. "I'll recommend you to someone, if you don't trust me," he said. He gave me the name of a woman gynecologist on the east side of Tucson. We lived on the west side, a good twenty miles away. I wondered why he could not recommend a gynecologist closer to our home. But he had achieved his purpose with the suggestion that I did not trust him. Of course, you trust your doctor. I never made an appointment with the gynecologist, who likely was another doctor in the holistic network. I decided that Dr. Jim undoubtedly had already spoken with her, and I would not have learned anything new.

I didn't realize how completely in bondage I had become to this new medical practice and the doctor who controlled it. Far be it from me to risk his disfavor by his thinking I didn't *trust* him.

Finally, Bud and I talked to Dr. Jim about adopting. We knew we would need a doctor's statement, certifying that we were in good health, to get state approval for adoption. He favored the adoption idea, even offering to keep his eyes open if an unmarried, pregnant patient, who wished to place her baby through private adoption, came into the clinic. "Obstetrics," he said, "is Dr. Mary's [his wife's] specialty."

Eventually, we learned a baby had become available. During my routine checkup, Dr. Jim mentioned that one of the clinic's woman patients had given birth to a healthy baby boy the day before. She wished to place the baby through private adoption. Were we interested? We were very interested but uncertain about the legal procedures. I said we would have to contact and consult with a lawyer first. Before we had time to contact a lawyer, however, we received a phone call the next morning from the clinic with the news: "The mother has decided to keep her baby."

After that, Dr. Jim occasionally inquired whether we still wanted to find a baby. We always said, "Of course," but no more babies were offered.

Later on, after we left the clinic and reflected on these incidents, we wondered: if we had been more worldly wise and had offered our doctor five or ten thousand dollars "under the table," would we have had more success adopting a child?

In 1974, I suffered from repeated upper respiratory and bladder infections, as well as mouth canker sores that took weeks to heal. Dr. Jim suggested I have a complete medical exam, including blood tests and an EKG.

Later, he reported, "The blood tests reveal anemia, and a photomotogram shows low thyroid activity." His treatment: two "natural remedies" dispensed by the clinic's pharmacy. One was Iron Plus, an iron tablet; the other was atomidine, a product of iodine trichloride, based on Edgar Cayce's readings for low thyroid activity. "Take the atomidine in a glass of water—one drop on Monday, two drops on Tuesday, and so on for five days. None on Saturday or Sunday; then start over again the following week."

I recalled my mother being treated similarly for low thyroid function with iodine drops, so it seemed reasonable that I too suffered this ailment. Dr. Jim quickly pointed out that the Midwest, where I'd grown up, is considered the "thyroid belt" of America. "Because landlocked Midwesterners don't eat much seafood containing natural iodine, they are more prone to thyroid problems," he said. He neglected to mention that with the advent of iodized salt, thyroid deficiencies were rare and no longer were being treated with iodine drops.

After taking Iron Plus daily for a year, with periodic blood counts, Dr. Jim announced my blood count was "okay," and I could discontinue the iron tablets. "If you start feeling fatigued again," he advised, "come in and get another bottle."

On several occasions I did purchase another bottle, but I often forgot to take them on schedule.

As the patient load at the clinic increased, it became harder to get an appointment with Dr. Jim without scheduling the appointment weeks in advance. Most of my appointments with him seemed to be of an emergency or sudden-illness nature, such as bladder infections. The clinic solved their doctor shortage by hiring licensed nurse practitioners (LNPs) and physician's assistants (PAs) to prescreen patients, as well as hiring holistic homeopathic doctors. Only the most serious medical cases received the attention of Dr. Jim or Dr. Mary.

"Don't you want me as your patient anymore?" I asked Dr. Jim on one rare medical visit with him. I had been very insistent that I didn't want to see anyone but him.

Dr. Jim acted genuinely hurt by my suggestion. He explained that the nurse practitioners and physician's assistants could attend to routine medical problems, such as: upper respiratory and bladder infections, flu, and gynecological exams. "By employing LNPs and PAs, the clinic is able to keep medical costs down for our patients," he explained.

Earlier, he had introduced me to Betty Miller, a licensed family nurse practitioner (FNP) who, he said, was a trained specialist in gynecological procedures. He urged me to use her for my yearly pelvic and pap tests. "She can better relate to you from a woman's point of view."

Just as Dr. Jim was a grandfatherly type, Betty seemed to be a completely trustworthy grandmotherly type—friendly, slightly plump, and gray-haired.

During my first pelvic exam, Betty explained what she was doing and why, in great detail. She was gentle and even warmed the speculum before inserting it. I liked Betty immediately. She had a wonderful bedside manner. Dr. Jim encouraged me to request Betty for all my medical prescreenings. In 1976, Betty essentially became my primary care physician.

I continued to experience monthly menstrual discomfort, now with increased frequency and severity. The castor oil packs no longer provided relief. Betty suggested that endometriosis might be the problem, a thought that had also crossed my mind after reading articles on the subject in women's magazines.

"Endometriosis," she explained, "can also cause infertility."

Bud and I still hoped for a mid-life pregnancy, and the clinic encouraged these hopes.

"There is no cure for endometriosis short of surgery," Betty advised, quickly suggesting, "You don't want to have surgery, do you?" She also counseled that if left untreated, endometriosis would dry up and disappear with menopause, when the menses ceased.

From my own reading, I knew endometriosis happened when the lining of the uterus wandered outside the uterus and into the abdominal cavity, where it attached itself to other pelvic organs. Betty reassured me, "It's usually a benign condition." (This seemed to imply I didn't have to worry about cancer.)

"With menopause," Betty clarified, "the lining of the uterus dries up and shrivels. The endometriosis, like tiny mini-uteruses, also dries up and shrivels. If you can stand the monthly pain, it will all be over in a few years, along with your periods." She planted her seeds well. Who wanted to have surgery, unless you needed it to save your life? "Having endometriosis doesn't necessarily mean a woman can't bear children," Betty said, explaining she had undergone surgery for endometriosis, yet she had borne four children—before her surgery. Like dangling a carrot in front of a mule, she nourished my hope, the hope of pregnancy, the hope of a baby.

I'd heard of many cases of "menopausal babies"—women who became pregnant, some with their first baby, during the pre-menopausal stage. One of my friends had her first and only baby at age forty. I was only thirty-eight, the same age as my mother when she had her *last* baby. My grandmothers both had their last children at age forty-three. It certainly was possible that I could have a menopausal baby.

As I grew older, I experienced heavier monthly bleeding. Betty assured me this probably meant early menopause—nothing to worry about. She reiterated that the pain would go away with menopause. She always encouraged me to believe this. And, trusting her, I did.

During some pelvic exams, Betty said she had removed "polyps" from the cervix, which were causing the between-period bleeding.

"A routine occurrence at your age," she said. She never suggested cancer. How could I know if she even removed any polyps?

Dryness of the vagina, diagnosed as a hormonal deficiency, received treatment with prescription estrogen creams. When a pap smear indicated low estrogen levels, she prescribed oral estrogen tablets.

In 1979, following my constant complaints of fatigue, Betty ordered blood tests, which she said showed anemia again. She blamed it on my heavy monthly periods and prescribed over-the-counter iron pills, along with prescription thyroid tablets and an assortment of vitamins, including calcium, and vitamins C and E. For a while, she scheduled follow-up visits, but progress lagged in resolving the anemia. I continued taking the iron, believing it would eventually combat my fatigue. Sometimes she prescribed two iron tablets if my counts dropped lower than normal. I began to take an interest in my hemoglobin counts, which usually were around 12.0, the lower edge of normal, and which indicated a tendency toward anemia. But Betty insisted the counts should be higher. I tried to eat more iron-rich foods, including liver at least once or twice a week.

In June 1979, I had a *severe* attack of pain, worse than normal. If it had been on the right side, I might have suspected appendicitis. I called the clinic for an appointment. Betty's schedule was full, so a male physician's assistant saw me. Besides menstrual cramps, I often suffered severe constipation and had not had a bowel movement for several days. I couldn't sit, I couldn't stand, and I couldn't walk without pain.

Charlie, the PA, performed a rectal exam and checked my stool for blood. There was none. But during the exam, he touched an extremely painful spot. I almost leaped off the exam table. He blamed my pain on constipation and advised me to take a well-known children's laxative— one teaspoonful every hour until I had a bowel movement. Before I left, the clinic scheduled an appointment for me with Betty the next day.

It took seventeen teaspoons of the laxative. Finally, seventeen hours later I had a bowel movement, and the pain lessened. The next day, Betty performed a routine pelvic exam, reporting "nothing out of the ordinary," although her diagnosis on my billing sheet showed "suspected ovarian cyst" and "possible endometriosis." Yet neither diagnosis prompted her to refer me to a gynecologist for follow-up treatment.

I had been led to believe that water cysts come and go, that they pose no serious problems. Betty's remedy to avoid future constipation incidents was, "Continue the children's laxative. It's made from natural ingredients and will not harm your intestinal tract." Her advice, as I later learned, was just another inaccurate piece of medical information.

Leafing through my thick medical folder, she reported that Dr. Jim had suspected endometriosis back in 1973.

"Why didn't he tell *me*?" I questioned. "He never mentioned endometriosis to me." For the first time, a note of suspicion crept into my mind. Never once had Dr. Jim mentioned that endometriosis might be the cause of my infertility, even though infertility was one of the reasons we were consulting him. *Could it have been corrected way back then*? I wondered.

Betty shrugged her shoulders; she didn't know why I hadn't been told *six years ago.*

Now, in addition to monthly menstrual pain, I had regular constipation and occasionally painful breasts, diagnosed as cystic breast disease, another benign condition, Betty said. No mammogram ever confirmed or refuted the cystic breast diagnosis.

Years before, while taking birth control pills, I complained of breast soreness. Dr. Jim sold me a breast salve, which reminded me of the bag balm my dad used on our cows when they had mastitis, an inflammation of the udder. It had helped the cows; perhaps it would help me.

Like the menstrual pain, the breast tenderness disappeared each month. I thought I was getting good medical care while avoiding dangerous, unnecessary prescription drugs and surgery. Who wants to have surgery? It didn't occur to me that I was now taking two prescription drugs—estrogen and thyroid pills. Were they dangerous and unnecessary? Yes, dangerous because they were both unnecessary.

I trusted Dr. Jim and his representatives. They always had plausible answers to my questions. When doubts arose, they always reassured me. Besides, I reasoned, the State Medical Association would not have referred me to a medical quack, would they? (The medical board can't know who the quacks are unless someone reports them.)

It is so easy to avoid noticing the things we do not want to see. And it is so easy to believe the words of assurance we want to hear.

CHAPTER 4

THE HOLISTIC BUBBLE BURSTS

In May 1981, I lost ten pounds in one month for no apparent reason. With my slight build, I could ill afford to lose that much weight on a regular basis. I remembered a similar rapid weight loss just before being diagnosed as "diabetic" in 1964, so I called the clinic, explained my weight loss, and suggested I have a complete blood count (CBC) taken to determine if my diabetes was "out of control" again. Although usually religiously strict about keeping to my diabetic diet, occasionally I slipped and indulged in sweets. Had I overindulged? It wouldn't hurt to check. Betty agreed and ordered the tests. When the results came back, she telephoned.

"Your hemoglobin count is *quite low* again," she said. "Why don't you come into the office so we can discuss the results?" I made an appointment.

My hemoglobin count was 11.4; the low normal is 12.0.

"A normal hemoglobin count for a woman your age," Betty explained, "is 13.5. You're *well below* normal." She sounded quite concerned, so I felt concerned too. "You're taking two 200-milligram iron tablets a day now," she stated, checking my file.

"No," I corrected her, "I'm only taking one tablet. I take it in the morning with my juice." I had been told to take one in the afternoon too, with supper, but I seldom remembered to take it.

"I want you to start taking *three* tablets a day."

"Can I take them all at the same time? Otherwise, I forget to take the later doses."

Betty agreed that all three tablets could be taken in the morning with my juice. "I also want to start you on weekly iron and liver shots," she added. I nodded mute agreement. After all, I paid my doctor to make these medical decisions for me. "We'll reevaluate you after a month." That was a new twist—she planned to *follow up* treatment.

After a month on tablets and shots, my blood count advanced from 11.4 to 11.6—a weak 0.2 increase. Betty, not ecstatic, suggested we continue for another month and reevaluate.

At the end of the second month, my hemoglobin advanced to 12.2, a jump of more than a half point. Encouraged, Betty suggested we continue the treatment for yet another month. At the end of the third month, my hemoglobin count dropped to 12.0. It was going in the *wrong* direction.

Because the iron therapy did not seem to be working, I expressed concern. "What is causing the anemia?" I asked. "We're only treating symptoms. What is *causing* it?"

Betty admitted she didn't know but pointed to my previous record of recovery. "You just have a very stubborn case," she said.

So it was my body's fault that recovery was slow.

Physically, I felt worse than ever. My energy level peaked by ten o'clock in the morning; whereas previously I could work until noon before tiring. I spent much of my day reading and generally taking it easy.

In 1970, I had given up my job as an advertising copywriter, hoping that if I showed I could be a stay-at-home mother, it would increase our chances for adoption. In the 1970s, however, young unmarried mothers often chose to keep their babies instead of putting them up for adoption. Supposedly, babies to adopt were in short supply.

Tucson had an unusually hot summer that year, not particularly conducive to vigorous activity, so I blamed my lack of pep and energy on the weather.

Breathing also became a problem. "It seems at times I cannot get enough air," I complained to Betty. I found myself breathing heavily, almost to the point of panting, after only mild exertion.

Betty always had a quick answer. Attempting to dismiss my fears, she said, "Your lungs are probably not getting enough oxygen. The red blood cells carry oxygen to the body. Your body is being starved for oxygen. When we get your blood count back up to normal, the other problem will also be resolved." Her explanations always had just enough of a ring of truth to make them sound plausible.

"I'm going to add vitamin B12 to your shot," she said, "to see if that helps."

I knew B12 treated pernicious anemia and hoped I didn't have *that*. I'd heard that people with pernicious anemia sometimes had to eat raw liver. While I liked liver, I didn't think I could stomach eating it raw. Betty also suggested I start taking vitamin E again and vitamin C—in large doses—and a vitamin B12 complex, in addition to the multivitamins and calcium pills I already took. I literally started each day with a handful of pills; most were taken in the morning so I wouldn't forget them later in the day. And now, weekly B12, "liver and iron" shots were added to the mix. (I'm sure the "liver and iron" shots were just another name for iron shots.)

I felt better after the first B12 shot. My energy level, though low, extended past lunchtime. I was grateful for that and tried to get more housework done.

Much later, I learned that vitamin B12 is a "feel good" vitamin. It gives a euphoric sense of well-being but quickly passes out of the body through the urinary tract. Now, I noticed that when I became tired I was exhausted. At night I sank into bed, totally drained. Even though I slept on a very firm mattress because of the arthritis in my back, when I lay down at night, I felt like a soft cloud was swallowing me. I floated down, down, down into its comfort. I didn't want to move. I didn't want to think. I didn't even want to breathe. I just wanted to *sleep*.

Sleep washed over me like a gentle fog. I slept the sleep of the dead, yet I always awoke feeling tired.

After a month on B12, and "liver and iron" shots, my hemoglobin advanced to a high 12.5. But then I experienced mental fuzziness. It was hard to describe, but the feeling seemed to affect my vision. At times, I felt like I was looking through a dirty window or a sheet of plastic film. The world around me appeared blurred and out of focus, yet when I blinked rapidly and concentrated hard, everything became clear. *I must be looking through the split in my bifocals*, I thought, dismissing the problem by blaming it on my inability to adjust to my new eyeglasses, although I'd worn them for more than a year. I rationalized away my symptoms. *It takes some people longer to adjust than others.*

My mind no longer felt sharp and alert. "Spaced out" is the term teenagers might use to describe the sensation. And no matter how long I slept, I always awoke feeling I still needed an extra hour or two of rest. Some days I even fell asleep in the afternoon. Since age four, I could never nap during daylight hours unless I was sick. But now, when I sat down to read, the words danced on the page. I'd close the book for a minute to rest my eyes and clear my head, only to find I'd been sleeping sitting up, sometimes for an hour or more. Never before had I been able to sleep while sitting up.

When this mental fuzziness struck, my brain felt slowed down; it felt almost *numb*. My concentration and memory were impaired. Often I found myself rubbing my forehead to restore circulation. If my lungs were starved for oxygen, perhaps my brain was starved too.

When I mentioned the mental fogginess to Betty, she dismissed it as sinus blockage and suggested an over-the-counter medication. I had a history of sinus and upper respiratory infections, but this was unlike any case I could remember. Betty refused to listen to my protest or consider anything else. "What else could it be?" she asked.

How should I know? I thought. *I'm not a doctor.*

Holistic medicine subtly shifts health care responsibility to the patient but without providing the necessary medical knowledge or training.

The conversation returned to my anemia and lack of progress. As if to justify her stand that I simply had a "stubborn case," Betty leafed through my thick medical file until she found an old CBC taken while I was still under Dr. Jim's care.

"Your blood count was only 11.0 then, lower then than it is now," she reported triumphantly.

"Then, why," I asked suspiciously, "am I taking *iron shots*? I never had to take shots before, and I got over it okay." (At least I thought I had.) I wondered if the shots were in some way aggravating my condition.

She quickly defended her treatment. "The shots get the iron into your system faster. Didn't you say you had more pep?"

"Yes, I did say that after the B12 addition," I admitted.

At the time I didn't understand the placebo effect—I wanted so much for my treatment to work that I'd convinced myself it *was* working.

"How much longer do I have to take these shots?" I asked. Logic told me that after four months there had to be a time limit, especially if they weren't helping.

"I'd like to see you take them until your hemoglobin reaches at least 13.5," Betty replied. That was one whole point away—if I didn't backslide. Maybe I could reach the "magic number" next month, September 1981, when I planned to visit my parents in Wisconsin and attend the wedding of my niece, Carole.

"Do you think I can go two weeks without a shot?" I asked.

"No, you can't. We can prepare a syringe for you to take along. Someone in your mother's doctor's office can inject it for you." As an afterthought, she added, "While you're there, why don't you check to see if anemia runs in your family?" It sounded like a reasonable request.

She sent the syringe of iron with me. My mother's doctor injected it. When I queried my family members about anemia, no one knew of any cases, but I learned my paternal grandfather had had leukemia when he died at age ninety-three. I later reported these findings to Betty.

"How high is my white count?" I asked.

She assured me, "Your white count is normal, but just to be on the safe side, why don't you come in for another CBC?" The white count measured 5.6, the low edge of normal but not indicative of leukemia. However, the hemoglobin had slipped to 11.9, despite our precautions to avoid skipped dosages. I had regressed to square one in the anemia game.

The week after I returned from my vacation, I planned to attend a regional women's church convention at Asilomar State Park in Pacific Grove, California. As editor of the group's newsletter, I needed to attend. The trip involved a sixteen-hour (all night) bus ride to the Asilomar convention grounds. On the morning of the day we left, I got an iron shot—"to give me energy for the week," I joked.

As soon as we arrived at the convention center in the morning, I dashed to an executive board meeting for the finalization of convention duties. The long meeting continued past my usual lunch hour. Combined with a sleepless night on the bus and an extra early breakfast on the road, my energy reserves were very low.

"If I don't get something to eat fast, I'm going to faint," I commented to a fellow board member when we finally broke for lunch. When I stood up to leave, I felt dizzy and oddly lightheaded. Mental calculations told me that more than six hours had passed since I'd eaten. I knew my blood sugar dropped rapidly after the sixth hour without food. Since experiencing the hypoglycemic reaction, I always secretly feared the possibility of this happening again. Lack of sugar in my system could easily be resolved by eating. What if I couldn't communicate this need?

I hurried to the dining hall but couldn't find the person with the meal tickets. Panic griped me. I fought to remain conscious and coherent.

For a convention filled to capacity with caring women, I saw no one to ask for help. *Everyone must be inside having lunch*, I thought, and without a meal ticket, I would be turned away. I sat on the outside steps of the dining hall, cradled my head in my arms, and started to cry. *I need help, Lord, immediately.* But no help came. *Where is everyone?* I felt like the proverbial starving man sitting on the steps of the banquet hall.

Finally, someone walked by. Seeing my difficulty, she asked if she could help. My breathing had become labored. Between deep breaths and sobs, I said, "I'm hypoglycemic. ... I need food ... immediately. ... Can't find the registrar. ... She has my lunch ticket."

The woman hurried to find the registrar after first offering me her lunch ticket while she searched. I declined her offer, uncertain if I could walk into the dining hall unassisted.

Soon other women gathered around me. One, a member of my home congregation and a retired registered nurse, offered me crackers from her purse. She carried them, she explained, for her diabetic husband.

The crackers temporarily brought me out of the reaction. Soon, I had a lunch ticket. Now that I was able to walk into the dining hall unassisted, I prayed for a short lunch line. No one was in line.

After eating, I felt stronger and more in control of my body, but I still was mentally foggy and physically shaky. The attack had all the outward appearances of an acute hypoglycemic reaction, yet something deep inside me nagged, *Could it be the anemia? Could this have something to do with the iron shots?*

Two days later, after walking in low heels on the retreat ground's hilly terrain, I noticed red spots under my big toenails on both feet. *Is it blood?* I wondered. *God, are you giving me a sign, trying to tell me I need to learn more about anemia—what causes it and what it causes?* I switched to flat shoes, and the condition grew no worse during the remaining two days.

By the end of the week, I felt stronger and more energetic. I knew my Christian friends were holding me up in prayer. From their concerned comments, I guessed word of my "attack" outside the dining hall had spread throughout the convention. (As editor of the district newsletter, everyone knew me by name, if not by sight.)

The long ride home robbed me of energy once again. I returned to Arcadia Clinic for another shot to help me recuperate. I seemed to *need* the shots and wondered vaguely if a person could become addicted to iron.

I continued to experience hypoglycemic reactions, even shortly after eating. All my nerves felt on edge, a typical hypoglycemic symptom but unusual for me. I had been a controlled hypoglycemic for sixteen years. I decided that something must be terribly wrong with my body.

Two weeks later, on my way to a neighborhood shopping center, one of the fuzzy episodes occurred. Although my eyesight and the part of my brain that controlled my senses felt muddled, my thinking processes remained entirely rational.

Dear God, I implored, *what am I doing out here on the street? In this condition, I'm a menace behind the wheel!*

As long as traffic moved in an easy-flowing orderly rhythm, I could follow it, robot-like. But if I needed to take unexpected, evasive action to prevent an accident, like putting on the brakes suddenly, I knew my brain could not process the information through my eyes to my hands or my feet quickly enough to brake or turn to avoid a collision. With such slowed reflexes, I was an accident waiting to happen.

Shaking my head rapidly sometimes cleared the cobwebs and sharpened my world, but on this day, nothing helped. I pulled into the nearest parking lot and rubbed my forehead and eyes—hard—in an effort to restore circulation. I remembered a similar incident when I had repeated that gesture on my vacation a month before. *I'm rubbing my forehead too much lately,* I thought, *and it's not helping. I need to learn more about anemia.*

On my way home, I stopped at a branch library. The card catalog listed only one book about anemia: Lawrence Galton's *The Disguised Disease: Anemia.*[3] Thankfully, I found it on the shelf. That afternoon and evening, I read most of the book.

For months I had asked Betty—and everyone else who I thought might know the answer—how long I should continue to take iron shots

---

[3] Lawrence Galton, *The Disguised Disease: Anemia* (New York: Crown Publishers, Inc., 1975).

without seeing some positive results. No one gave me a straight answer. Betty's pat answer was, "As long as you need them."

Logic told me there *had* to be a time limit—and there is. Galton pointed out that if a person's hemoglobin count had not risen two points after three months of iron treatment (from 11.4 to 13.4, in my case), the patient should be referred to a hematologist for further evaluation. Lawrence Galton is a medical journalist, the author of 22 books. Galton didn't recommend iron shots at all. With modern medical improvements, iron could be adequately absorbed in the body in pill form, he stated. With regard to vitamin B12, Galton said a person should be referred to a hematologist after one month without a two-point increase.

I was furious with rage. I had taken iron shots for five months and in combination with B12 for three months. My next shots were scheduled for the next day; I decided to ask Betty for a referral.

As I sat in the waiting room, Betty breezed in. Spotting me, she stopped for a minute and asked warmly, "How are you feeling?"

"I think I need to see a hematologist," I said evenly, holding up Galton's book. "I've been reading up on anemia."

She flitted out of the room to get the name and address of a hematologist that the clinic "often used." She returned and handed me a slip of paper, remarking, "You can try him, but I'm sure you won't learn anything new. Your white count is fine."

White count? I thought. *What does that mean? What does that have to do with anything? Could she be trying to talk me out of seeing a hematologist?* The thought flickered briefly in my mind, but I dismissed it. *You'd think she'd welcome another opinion since she obviously is having no success in getting to the root of my problem.*

The name on the slip of paper was for a doctor of osteopathy (DO). I'd expected to receive the name of a medical doctor hematologist. At that time, MDs and DOs didn't refer patients to each other. Arcadia Clinic hired only MDs—or so I'd thought when I became their patient.

"Will you let me know what you find out?" Betty asked sweetly, expressing concern for my welfare.

I promised I would. But the more I thought about her comment that I wouldn't learn *anything new*, the angrier I became. Suddenly, I knew what was really upsetting me. I didn't trust her anymore. And I didn't trust the osteopathic doctor to whom she referred me—someone, I suspected, who had no more knowledge or competence than she had. Did doctors cover up for one another? I didn't know. What I *did* know was that I didn't have to accept Betty's recommendation.

I called the Arizona Medical Association's doctor referral number and asked for the name of a hematologist in my area. Then I called Dr. Victor Fields and made an appointment for the following Friday.

At Dr. Fields's request, I asked Betty for copies of all my blood work, which, I suddenly realized, went back eight years to when Dr. Jim had begun treating me for anemia—*eight long, tired, anemic years.*

Betty gave me the lab reports in a sealed envelope—I suspected that the contents were not meant for my eyes. But the sealed envelope had my name on it and beckoned me to open it, which I did. I charted all the information from the CBCs, and an interesting pattern emerged.

At no time in my eight years of treatment did I *ever* have a normal hemoglobin count of 13.0 or higher, as Dr. Jim had suggested when he said I could discontinue treatment because "everything is okay." Eight years ago, *both* the red and white cell counts were below normal. While under Dr. Jim's care for anemia, my highest hemoglobin recorded was 12.0. It showed 12.0 when I began iron treatment and it was at the same 12.0 level when he said I could discontinue the iron tablets. In the year intervening, it had dipped to a low 10.8. No one ever suggested that I consult a hematologist to learn the reason for this erratic hemoglobin count.

The type of red blood cells noted in all my CBCs was "normochromic, normocytic"—normal in size, shape, and color, although deficient in numbers.

Any doctor with a modicum of knowledge about anemia would have known that I did *not* have iron deficiency anemia—and I never did.

Iron deficiency anemia is characterized by hypochromic (pale color), microcytic (small size) red cells. Pernicious anemia, which is treated with B12, is usually characterized by hyperchromic (bright red color) and macrocytic (large size) red cells.

Normochromic, normocytic cells, I learned later, are found in hemolytic anemia—the anemia of chronic disease, the type of anemia found in many patients with cancer, particularly lymphoma and leukemia, as well as diseases of the autoimmune system, such as rheumatoid arthritis, lupus, and multiple sclerosis.

Why didn't either Dr. Jim or Betty know that? What was I paying them for? I should have been referred to a hematologist months—*years*—ago. Treatment had already been delayed eight years. *Dear God*, I wondered, *at what price?*

CHAPTER 5

"YOUR MEDICINE IS DOING YOU NO GOOD"

On Friday, October 30, 1981, the nurse ushered me into Dr. Fields's office. In one hand I carried a large plastic bag containing the medications and vitamins I currently took. In the other hand, I carried an envelope with the photocopied CBC reports from Arcadia Clinic that Dr. Fields had requested I bring. The envelope also contained a file folder with the CBC summary I had prepared and a long list of questions.

Dr. Fields took one look at my CBC summary, glanced at the photocopied reports from the clinic, and said emphatically, "Stop taking *everything* you are now taking. Don't take any more iron shots. Don't take any more iron tablets. Don't take the vitamins or the Entozyme [a stomach enzyme Betty had prescribed to get the iron into my system faster]. You do not have iron deficiency anemia. Your medicine is doing you no good."

"Then why," I asked, puzzled, "did I feel so energized after getting the shots if they weren't doing me any good?"

He sighed and patiently tried to explain. "B12 can give you a sense of well-being." His words suggested that the shots gave me no actual energy; they just made me *think* they did. In medical circles, this is known as the placebo effect. A person wants so much to feel better that he or she does feel better—for a time. That explained the exhaustive fatigue after each short-lived recovery; I was burning up energy reserves I didn't have.

"Do I even have anemia?" I questioned, wondering if I had been led down a primrose path of pricey shots and costly clinic visits. *How many vitamin companies does Betty own stock in?* I wondered bitterly.

"According to your CBCs, you are anemic," Dr. Fields confirmed. "I suspect a lazy bone marrow"—my bone marrow simply did not produce enough red cells—"so for you, anemia might be a normal condition." He wanted to do a complete physical exam and bone marrow test to confirm his diagnosis. I wanted to get to the bottom of my mysterious anemia problem once and for all. I readily consented to the tests.

During the course of the physical exam, he noticed the red blood accumulated under my toenails. "A recent development," I told him. "I didn't drop anything on my toes."

"When did you have your last pelvic and pap smear?"

"Four months ago. I usually have it done around my birthday in June."

"Did you go to a gynecologist?"

"No, Betty, the family nurse practitioner at Arcadia Clinic, did it. She's specially trained in gynecology and qualified to do that," I said, parroting what I had been told. "She told me all the tests were normal, other than once when she reported my estrogen level was 'quite low.' I've been taking estrogen tablets for just over a year."

"I think you should see a gynecologist. Do you know one?"

"No, but I can ask a friend." I hated finding a new doctor—a doctor I could trust.

"Your breasts are quite cystic. Have you ever had a mammogram?"

"I *know* I have cystic breast disease. I've had it for years. But no, I never had a mammogram. Betty didn't think it was necessary."

"Do they hurt?" he queried, "Are they tender to touch?"

"Yes, they're often quite sore, especially just before my period."

"I don't think you need to take the estrogen either," he said.

"How about the thyroid?" I asked. "Betty told me once you start taking thyroid medicine, you have to take it every day for the rest of your life—that you shouldn't stop taking it abruptly."

"You can take the thyroid medication," he said. He took a complete history and then asked, "Is there cancer in your family?"

"My mother's aunt died from breast cancer, and my grandfather had leukemia when he died at age ninety-three. Other than that, none that I know of."

He wanted the mammogram done at once and scheduled a Wednesday appointment. Dr. Fields performed the bone marrow test that day in a special sterile room in his suite of offices.

A local anesthetic deadened the area for the bone marrow sample. While I lay face down on a specially designed table for this procedure, the doctor inserted a large-bore needle into my left hip bone, the side where all the pain was localized. I felt only pressure during the procedure; it was no more painful than a tooth extraction, with minimal bleeding. He dressed the puncture wound with a sterile bandage. After a few minutes, he let me sit up.

Dr. Fields, already preparing slides, showed me the bone marrow he had extracted. It rested in a capped bottle of special solution, preparatory for shipment to another lab for further testing. The core, about an inch long, was about the size of the little straws packaged with boxed juices, sponge-like in texture and bone-gray in appearance. It looked just as I would have expected bone marrow to look.

Although Dr. Fields warned I might feel weak for a while afterward, I felt fine and had no trouble swinging my legs off the table, walking, or driving myself home. The hip felt numb. As the anesthetic wore off, however, I experienced some pain and tenderness. I wished I had not scheduled a yard sale with my neighbor for the next two days.

Acutely aware of the puncture area, I tried to avoid bumping it. I sat gingerly, balancing my weight on my good hip. Still, it did not interfere with normal activities. Walking didn't hurt, although I favored the punctured hip for several days and walked with a slight limp. A week later, only a vague, dull ache remained to remind me of the test.

A few days after the bone marrow test, I had a mammogram. The female technician helped put me at ease. It seemed that my breasts were x-rayed from every conceivable angle: top, bottom, sides. At times, when she tried to flatten the breast tissue to get a better picture, I thought she might pinch them off, but she never actually pinched them. I was not uncomfortable during this procedure, though I had heard other women complain about this test. As she removed the negative plates from the developer, I noticed large white spots in my breasts. *Are those the cysts?*

She told me that a staff doctor wanted to see me, and a short, slightly built man walked into the room. "Do you mind if I check your breasts?" he asked.

It surprised me to hear him ask permission; but was pleased that he did. Obviously, this doctor understood the sensitive feelings of his female patients. I consented, assuming he needed to check for something specific. I wanted the problem resolved. I had lived with uncertainly and anxiety far too long.

He thoroughly palpitated the breast tissue and checked for lumps under my armpits. He worked quickly, without comment, and finished in less than five minutes. The results, he said, would be reported to Dr. Fields.

Dr. Fields called about a week later with all the test results. The mammogram showed no abnormalities. The breasts, although cystic, showed no signs of tumors or cancerous growths.

The bone marrow exam, however, contradicted his initial diagnosis of a lazy bone marrow. "Yours," he stated, "is highly cellular—plenty of red blood cells are being produced, but for some unexplained reason not yet clear, the cells are being destroyed in your system." He named two different types of abnormal cells found in my bone marrow, but he assured me they were not found in large quantities. "It might mean nothing. Many people have abnormal cells that creep in from time to time," he counseled, "or they could be the early indication of a problem."

Later, as I studied hematology, I noted that the abnormal cell types he mentioned were associated with bone cancers.

My platelet count in the mid-normal range, about 250,000, was a healthy sign. Had it been low, that might have explained the under-toenail bleeding. With a low platelet count, blood is able to leak through the skin, causing easy bruising. I did bruise easily, but that didn't seem to be the reason. The sedimentation rate of forty (about twice as high as it should be) indicated infection or inflammation in my system, but it was not dangerously high.

"Make an appointment to see me again in three months," Dr. Fields advised, "unless you have problems." He didn't elaborate on what type of "problems" to expect. But he wanted to recheck my blood counts after more of the iron was out of my system.

In the meantime, I undertook a voracious reading program in hematology at the local public library. At my next visit with Dr. Fields, I would be knowledgeable about my condition so I could ask intelligent questions, keep track of meaningful symptoms, and hopefully help him to find the root cause of my problem.

The public library, sadly, lacked hematology books written in layman's language. I began a notebook of medical terms and their definitions, so whenever I encountered the word again, I could quickly double-check its meaning. After reading several scholarly volumes, I started to understand the medical terminology, referring to my notebook less and less often.

And I learned facts, information that, had I known eight years earlier, would have led me to change doctors sooner. The usual therapeutic dose of iron is 200 milligrams of oral iron a day. For best results, the dosage should be divided into two or more doses per day, separated by at least four hours. I took three tablets, each supplying 200 milligrams of iron—a total of 600 milligrams of iron daily—all taken at the same time, per Betty's instructions.

The iron tablets had been supplemented with weekly iron shots. Iron shots, I learned, can supply up to four times the normal therapeutic dose of iron, or 800 additional milligrams of iron. On the days I received shots, it was possible that my iron input topped 1,400 milligrams, seven times the daily therapeutic dose of iron.

In comparison, the National Research Council recommended 12

milligrams of iron daily for adults and 15 milligrams for adolescents and pregnant women. On some days, I probably received more than a hundred times the normal recommended daily dose of iron—and none of it needed because I did not have iron deficiency anemia. My body was being overdosed, poisoned with iron (and vitamins too, I learned later). While the doctors at Arcadia Clinic said they didn't believe in prescribing dangerous prescription drugs, it seemed they didn't mind poisoning their patients with over-the-counter drugs.

For years, my stools had been black and tarry, indicating iron overdose—or bowel cancer. Betty occasionally checked for blood with the Hemoccult test, assuring me there was no sign of blood and thus ruling out bowel cancer.

In 1975, research revealed the Hemoccult test results were invalid if a person took 500 milligrams or more of vitamin C within three days of the test. Vitamin C would cause the test to show a false negative reading, regardless of whether blood was present in the stool sample. I had been taking 500 to 1000 milligrams of vitamin C for years. Betty did not instruct me to discontinue taking it before the Hemoccult test. Her assurances of "no blood in your stool" showed her ignorance about how vitamin C could influence this test. *How could she know for sure there was no blood in my stool?* I wondered.

Iron, I learned, should *not* be taken orally if it's given by injection. Unneeded iron taken on a continuous basis can be hazardous to one's health, causing such problems as (1) hemochromatosis, a disorder in which iron becomes stored in the body's tissues and is characterized by a bronze discoloration of the skin (at least, my skin had not changed color); (2) diabetes (bingo—did it cause hypoglycemia too?); (3) impaired heart function; (4) liver damage; and (5) sexual impotence. I wondered how many women took iron tablets for fatigue without being tested, thinking iron couldn't harm them.

Additionally, ingestion of large amounts of iron is especially harmful to individuals with a predisposition toward rheumatoid arthritis. Researchers in England and the United States found that oral iron therapy aggravates conditions of early rheumatoid arthritis by contributing to joint inflammation; consequently, iron should be used cautiously whenever this type of arthritis is suspected.[4]

Dr. Jim knew I'd moved to Tucson from Minneapolis because rheumatoid arthritis was suspected as the cause of my back pain and was aggravated by the cold Minnesota winters.

Early in our doctor/patient relationship, Dr. Jim had changed my diagnosis from rheumatoid arthritis to osteoarthritis because no physical evidence indicated joint or bone deterioration.

Sardonically, I thought, *First doctors cause the disease, and then they try to cure it.* Could doctors really be so callous as to create long-term-care patients?

Besides tarry stools, iron overdose can also manifest itself in drowsiness, lethargy, extreme weakness, shallow breathing, and coma, to name just a few of the side effects. I experienced all those symptoms, except coma, although I might have come very close at the district women's convention.

Normachromic, normacytic anemias—the hemolytic anemias—are caused by cell destruction. Causes for this type of anemia can range from chronic infections, such as a sinus infection, to the dreaded cancers.

The difficult phase still lay ahead: finding the cause of my anemia.

---

[4] Lawrence Galton, "Iron Plus Arthritis Equals Trouble," *Family Circle*, January 4, 1983, 102.

CHAPTER 6

"DO YOU HATE ME?"

Betty had asked me to call her with the results of the hematologist's findings. Naively, I promised I would, so I thought it only fair that I should tell her about her medical ignorance, which, in a small way, might protect the next unsuspecting victim. (It never occurred to me that she coldly and calculatingly had deliberately planned those treatments to keep me as a long-term-care patient.)

The hematologist's report upset me; actually, livid and enraged might better describe my state of mind when I called the clinic asking to speak to Betty. "She's busy," the receptionist said. "She'll return your call at her earliest convenience."

She called at seven o'clock that night.

"What are the side effects of all this stuff you've been giving me all summer?" I calmly asked.

"I don't know," she replied lightly. "What are they?"

"You're the doctor," I countered, my voice now harsh with anger. "You prescribed it. You're supposed to know."

"I don't think I gave you anything that would harm you," she replied, a little too defensively.

"You don't *think*? Do you know? I got the results of the bone marrow test. They found abnormal cells, and the sedimentation rate is quite high, indicating infection."

"Maybe we looked into your problem just in time."

"*We?*" I spat the words into the telephone receiver. "*We?* Just tell me what *you* did. *You* didn't do anything. You didn't do your homework. *I* looked into it. *I* asked to be referred. You didn't think I'd learn anything new, remember? Would you *ever* have referred me if I hadn't asked? You don't even know enough to know when to refer. What did I pay you for? Sympathy?" *I have friends who can provide that service for free,* I thought reproachfully.

"I think you were just extra-concerned about your health when you learned about your grandfather's leukemia," she said, trying to soothe me and quell my anger.

"And it's a good thing I was. You certainly didn't seem concerned. You didn't take time to research my anemia, but you had plenty of time to run off to a workshop in Russia this summer." I stopped for a moment to let my words sink in before I dropped the clincher. "I don't have iron deficiency anemia." I spewed the words with all the venom of a person betrayed. "I never had it. The hematologist told me to quit taking everything—the iron, the vitamins, everything. I should have been referred to a hematologist after three months when the iron therapy didn't correct the problem and after one month when B12 didn't help. Do you even *know* that?"

"All doctors make mistakes," she said, lamely defending herself. "Even the best doctors make mistakes now and then."

Not with my body, they don't, I thought. *Not if they want to continue being my doctor.*

I should have reminded her that she was not a doctor, only a nurse practitioner who thought of herself as a doctor. But apparently she also remembered her status for she quickly said, "I don't make all these decisions by myself, you know. I consulted Dr. Mary."

"I know you *said* you consulted her," I replied, "and if you did, that doesn't give me any more confidence in Dr. Mary's ability as a doctor than it does in yours. Did you ever consult with Dr. Jim? Since he's the one who first treated me for anemia, it seems he's the one you should have consulted. Apparently, after a year's time, he realized the iron treatment didn't do any good; that's why he discontinued it. Did you ever discuss my anemia with him?"

How naive of me to think Dr. Jim was blameless.

"No," she admitted. "Dr. Jim hasn't been associated with the clinic in a medical capacity for many years."

Her statement came as news to me but didn't really surprise me. I knew Dr. Jim spent many hours fund-raising for the holistic medical association. Had Dr. Mary become the sole physician on the clinic's staff? As one of the founding members of the American Holistic Medical Association, she, too, seemed to spend much of her time touring and lecturing, extolling the virtues of this new health care concept. Was all the doctoring at Arcadia Clinic being handled by doctor's assistants and nurse practitioners with no physician oversight?

I recalled one Friday afternoon when I'd asked Betty a question she couldn't answer. "I'm sorry," she'd said. "No doctor is in the clinic today." Her admission about the *lack* of doctor/patient supervision dumbfounded me.

"How long would you have continued to give me iron shots?" I demanded. "How long? *Forever?*" I waited for her reply, but none was forthcoming. "I don't trust you anymore," I said evenly. My anger was spent. I hoped I had educated her about her medical ignorance. "My hematologist said that because of my cystic breasts, I should have had a mammogram years ago, if for no other reason than to use for comparison."

"Did you have a mammogram?"

"Yes."

"What did they find?"

"I have cystic breasts, but everything is okay."

"Why don't you come into the office next week? We'll talk—just you and me and Dr. Mary. We'll sit down and discuss your case. If you want, we'll assign you to a different doctor. We're getting a new one on the staff—"

"There's nothing for us to talk about," I interrupted. "I just wanted you to know that I plan to change doctors, and it won't be a holistic medical practitioner. I'll expect you to forward my medical files. I'll let you know where to send them."

Many times since, I have thanked God that I didn't take Betty's offer to come in and talk. Not until years later did I fully realize the deep psychological control holistic practitioners have over their patients. Had I returned for that conference, I might never have escaped the *unholy grip* holistic medicine held over me.

"I didn't do anything to deliberately hurt you." Betty's voice quavered. She sounded on the verge of tears. "Do you think I did? Do you hate me?"

What an odd question, I thought. Did I *hate* her? Did she think I should love her for her misdiagnosis and mistreatment? Why should she be concerned whether I hated her or loved her or cared about her at all? I didn't plan to see her ever again.

After a long pause, I replied, "No, I don't hate you. I feel sorry for you. You don't even know what you *don't* know. More than anything else I'm disappointed. I expected better. I trusted you. But you were too busy, running from symposium to workshop, to do your homework. You don't care about your patients."

More to be pitied than scorned, I thought as I hung up the receiver.

I never saw or heard from Betty again. I subscribed to the school of thought that teaches "Fool me once, shame on you; fool me twice, shame on me." Although I asked that my medical files be forwarded to my new doctor, they were never sent. Much later, I wondered if I should not have phoned her that day and vented my frustration. Had I unintentionally given her a "heads up," an opportunity to sanitize and destroy incriminating evidence in my medical files? I would never know.

Reflecting back on our conversation, I noticed similarities between what I saw happening in my holistic doctor's office and what I observed happening in our mega-church. The leaders, pastors, and lay professionals were so busy attending seminars and workshop—learning new insights, new approaches, new ways to handle old problems—they had neither the time nor the energy to communicate with parishioners or address their needs. Our pastors and church leaders had no time for ministry.

People with problems were not helped; they were ignored. All that mattered was learning new technologies, new theologies, and new ways to encourage congregational giving. A disproportionate amount of time was spent raising funds. What had happened to trusting God to supply all our needs?

My pastors, I thought, *have stopped* doing *the Word*.

CHAPTER 7

"YOUR TEST FOR LUPUS WAS SLIGHTLY POSITIVE"

The pain struck a few days before Christmas 1981, excruciating pain in the lower left side of my abdomen. When I experienced a similar painful incident in June 1979, Betty explained the pain might be caused by the swelling of endometrial tissue that had wandered outside the ovaries into the abdominal cavity, possibly causing some intestinal blockage. But she didn't think it was anything to be concerned about.

Usually, the worst pain occurred the first day or two of my menstrual flow. But this time, I was finished with my menses. It was not normal to be having menstrual pain a week later.

It was one of my worst-ever attacks of cramps. With no relief from using the castor oil packs, uncontrolled pain dominated my day. By the second day, I couldn't stand. I couldn't sit. I couldn't walk. I couldn't lie down. Pain reigned. No position offered relief. The ache was intense and constant. It started in the lower left abdomen, wrapped itself around my entire lower body, and radiated upward to my waist. Did it originate in the kidney area? The hip bone? The bowel? Where? It was all-encompassing. *Everything hurt.*

Finally, unable to stand the agony any longer, I gave myself an enema. It always had helped before, but not this time. Although the discomfort mimicked menstrual pain, it couldn't be menstrual pain; I wasn't menstruating. The pain intensified. By ten o'clock at night, convinced I'd never sleep with such an unrelenting ache, I asked my husband to call Dr. Fields's night number. I described my pain to the doctor on duty.

"You'd better go to the emergency ward at the hospital," he advised. "It could be appendicitis."

It isn't on the right side for appendicitis? I thought, but I recalled hearing of people whose appendix was located on the wrong side.

In the emergency ward, after an abdominal x-ray, the nurse gave me another enema. She had difficulty getting the enema started, although she said it appeared to be inserted correctly.

"I don't think there's anything left in my bowel to come out," I explained when the enema bag refused to empty. She persisted. Finally, she achieved success. As I predicted, my bowel was practically devoid of fecal material.

As the evening progressed, the pain subsided. Two hours later, I left the hospital with only a nagging ache. The doctor gave me a prescription for pain medication and a written recommendation to have the lower bowel examined by a proctologist.

I called Dr. Fields's office the next morning. He referred me to a proctologist. It hadn't even been two months since I first consulted him. *This must be one of the problems he warned me about*, I thought. *What does it all mean?* Still, I was happy to have finally found a doctor who would investigate and follow-up on the cause of my pain.

Betty always dismissed my late-night calls when I'd complained of pain, referring me to the "trusty castor oil pack" instead of to a specialist. Once the pain subsided—and fortunately, it always did—no one from my holistic medical team attempted to track down the cause. Their attitude seemed to be "out of sight, out of mind."

Dr. Winston, the proctologist, reported finding some hemorrhoid polyps but nothing to be concerned about. When I asked if the polyps could have caused the pain, he replied, "Hemorrhoids themselves don't cause pain."

I knew what he meant. Only inflamed or infected hemorrhoids cause pain. Apparently, mine were neither.

I returned to Dr. Fields, who ordered another battery of blood tests, including one for bone cancer. It encouraged me that he had finally decided to test for that. I continued to haunt the library, hoping to learn which problems were being eliminated.

In a few days, his nurse called with the test results, which were all normal—another dead end. She scheduled another appointment for me in three months.

The search for the cause of my anemia had covered five fruitless months by the time I met the hematologist for my third visit in March. I had accumulated hundreds of dollars' worth of blood tests, a bone marrow test, a mammogram, a rectal exam, and a sigmoidoscopy. Although we had eliminated many possibilities, we seemed no closer to an answer.

I began a diary of symptoms so I wouldn't forget some insignificant complaint that might be the key to diagnosis. My symptoms seemed diverse and unrelated: bone pain, especially in the left shin and left pelvic area; mild bone pain in the right forearm and entire rib cage; intermittent pain in the lung area, especially upon rising in the morning; breathing difficulties (sometimes I felt I would smother for lack of air); swollen lymph glands in the neck; difficulty swallowing, with a feeling of fullness or swelling under the tongue; lightheadedness and feelings of faintness, mostly in the evening before bedtime; and occasional nausea and dizziness.

Shortly before my March appointment, I accidentally bumped my left shin and a huge welt raised on it. It swelled much larger than it should have for such a slight bump. The welt only hurt when I pressed on it. Walking didn't cause pain, but sitting, especially with one leg crossed over the other, produced intense throbbing. I sat in my easy chair, legs elevated and uncrossed, trying to ignore the pain.

Holistic medical practitioners carefully condition their patients to ignore pain. This delays the process of their seeking real answers to medical complaints. As a good patient, I had learned the lesson well and often ignored pain.

Ten years earlier, I had fallen over backward while standing on a folding chair. My left leg got trapped between the wooden seat and metal bar at the back of the chair, pinching the shin so severely that a small indentation remained in my leg for months afterward. Had I damaged the bone or caused a deep bone bruise? I wondered. At the time, I didn't consult a doctor. It hadn't seemed necessary. The leg turned black and blue, but it didn't swell or show other signs of serious injury. Occasionally, it pained me in damp weather, which I attributed to the arthritis that had brought me to Arizona twenty years ago. Until now, I had completely forgotten about the shin injury.

I reported all these symptoms to Dr. Fields during my March appointment. He listened, taking notes without comment. Finally, he asked, "Have you ever noticed if you were photosensitive to the sun?"

"Yes," I replied, wondering what prompted that strange question. "One of the reasons I quit my job as a school crossing guard three years ago was because of a sun allergy."

At the time, my cheeks and nose turned bright red whenever exposed to the sun for long periods, especially in the afternoon as I waited to help the children cross the street. Weekends, when I was indoors, the rash faded. Weekdays, when I returned to my post in the sun, it brightened. The Arizona sun was hottest during my two-to-four-o'clock shift. Temperatures often reached 110 degrees in September, during the first weeks of school, and again in June, during the last weeks. There was no shade at my location. I wore a wide-brimmed hat to guard against skin cancer, but it did not completely block the sun's rays from my face.

I had mentioned the rash to Betty, wondering if it could be a sun allergy. She agreed it probably was. "If you are allergic to the sun, perhaps you should give up your school crossing-guard job," she recommended, and I complied. Once I quit and got out of the sun, I had no more facial rashes.

"In the last blood work, your test for lupus was slightly positive,"

Dr. Fields explained. "I want to rerun it with another test." He planned to order an ANA (antinuclear antibodies) test, plus a more definitive C-3 test (low levels of C-3 indicate active lupus). I nodded my assent.

Lupus—I didn't even know what that disease was, except that it was a fairly new ailment. I had seen advertisements for "Live with Lupus" meetings that taught patients how to live with this medical condition. I'd mastered living with diabetes. If necessary, I could learn to live with lupus too. *It's better than having cancer*, I thought.

Ever since I'd started reading hematology books, looking for a clue to the cause of my hemolytic anemia, cancer always lurked in the back of my mind. The library's reference section had become my second home, especially after Dr. Fields ordered new blood tests. If results came back normal, I wanted to know which problem had been eliminated. And if they didn't come back normal, I wanted to know which problem still needed to be confronted.

Unfortunately in 1981, my library research didn't always find and identify the blood tests being ordered.

I had stopped taking all the vitamins my holistic doctors had prescribed, but I still took the thyroid medication. Because I hadn't visited a gynecologist, I continued to take the estrogen tablets until December 1, about a month after my first appointment with Dr. Fields.

Now, he asked if I had seen a gynecologist yet.

"I haven't had any problems lately," I answered. "I thought I could wait." I hadn't considered the painful episode and emergency room visit in December to be gynecologically related.

"I want you to see a gynecologist right away," he insisted. "The x-rays taken at the hospital in December indicated calcium deposits in your abdomen. I can't make an accurate diagnosis until you've seen a gynecologist. Do you mind if I make an appointment for you? There's a good gynecologist in this building."

"Okay," I agreed. Dr. Fields, I was certain, would recommend the best. Everything he'd told me so far correlated with what I'd read in the library's hematology books. I was assured that he knew his business and felt he would not lead me astray. Finally, I had found a good doctor, one I could trust. And he wouldn't quit until he found the cause of my problem.

"You have an appointment with Dr. John Lance tomorrow morning at nine thirty," he said. "I discussed your case with him."

When I left the office, I hurried to my best friend—the public library—to research lupus. My college library science minor had become a godsend in helping me research.

Systemic lupus erythematosus (SLE) is characterized by a red butterfly-shaped rash on the nose and cheekbones—the same kind of unusual rash I noticed on my face when I worked as a school crossing guard. Lupus belongs to the rheumatoid arthritis family. Anemia and an elevated sedimentation rate were just a few of the symptoms. Others included chest pain; pain in the stomach, muscles, and joints; fatigue, weakness, chills, and low-grade fever.

Dear God, I thought, *I've had all these symptoms at some time, although the chills were usually accompanied by bladder infections*. I didn't have fluid retention in my feet or ankles, another symptom, but the chest discomfort—I suffered pleurisy-like pain in my lungs.

Lupus is caused by a defect in the body's defense mechanism; it's a chronic inflammation of the body's connective tissue. The immune system wages war against and destroys itself. Both heredity and environment play a role. The immune system destroys the good antibodies along with the bad ones, as if the body is unable to detect which antibodies to save and which to destroy. In that respect, it resembles the uncontrolled cell destruction of cancer. There was no known cause or cure for lupus.

Only recently was an accurate blood test developed to positively identify lupus patients. The symptoms are so similar to many other medical conditions, including heart and kidney disease, that SLE is often difficult to recognize and detect.

In addition, stress, injury, infection, and excessive exposure to sunlight can intensify lupus. But like arthritis, it can go into long periods of remission.

My arthritis had been in remission for almost fifteen years, since moving to Arizona. Now I wondered, did I ever have arthritis? Or was it undiagnosed lupus? Could the arthritis diagnosis that brought me to Arizona actually have been lupus? Twenty years ago, an accurate test for lupus wasn't yet developed.

I remembered that when I lived in Minneapolis I had taken iron tablets for symptoms of anemia. After three months, my doctor told me to discontinue taking the iron tablets, and I believed the anemia had been resolved. Did he realize that iron was not the solution to my anemia? I also remembered being told my blood sedimentation rate was high, although I couldn't remember how high.

Rheumatoid arthritis had been the diagnosis. The joint pain in my lower back had been extremely severe, especially in the cold, wet Minnesota winter months. A few years before, I'd been thrown from a horse and had landed on my back on a clump of frozen dirt. Back pain had developed after that incident. My doctor prescribed infrared heat treatments for several months. I spent an hour in the morning and an hour in the evening lying under a heat lamp, drying out my bones. Dr. McLeod warned that calcium deposits could "freeze" the hip joints, rendering them useless, unless I exercised regularly.

"When you feel the worst, you must move the most," he counseled. Finally, he recommended that I move out West to a warmer, dryer climate—Denver or Arizona.

By spring 1962, just months before my twenty-fourth birthday, I decided I was not living; I was only existing. I didn't want to spend the rest of my life lying under a heat lamp. My younger brother, Bert, had recently traveled to Arizona on a sales trip. He brought back tales of mild winters.

That summer I gave notice at work and looked forward to spending the next winter in warm, dry Arizona. In September, I left Minneapolis with a college friend, Helen, who also was looking for a change of scenery and new adventures after breaking up with her boyfriend. She owned a 1950 Chevy Powerglide. I took a summer AAA driver's education course, obtaining my learner's permit before we left. I could help drive. Neither of us would have to endure another freezing Minnesota winter.

We arrived in Tucson on September 12, 1962, expecting temperate fall weather. It was more than 110 degrees, and we didn't have air conditioning in the car. It was suffocatingly hot. I felt like someone had thrown a heavy blanket over me. Helen's hands were so sweaty that to combat the heat, she used Kleenex to hold onto the steering wheel when she drove.

"Let's just turn around and go back to Wisconsin," she said. Wisconsin was her home state.

I reminded her, "We promised to give it a year."

We found a cheap motel with a pool on the main drag through Tucson. Every day we cooled off in the pool. Finally, after a week, we decided we needed jobs. Helen found one first at a daycare center. Since I didn't have a car, I found a job as a copywriter and Girl Friday with a one-man advertising agency close enough to our new apartment that I could walk to work.

Inside of a year, Helen was married and expecting their first child. It took me five more years to find my husband, Bud.

In Arizona, my arthritis improved surprisingly quickly. That convinced me I had made the right decision to move out West.

Dr. Jim said, "There is no all-inclusive test to determine which type of arthritis you have." He thought I had osteoarthritis.

Now I wondered if I had arthritis at all. Whatever I had, it was in remission. Because I was no longer troubled with lower-back pain, I didn't really care if it was arthritis or something else.

On the other hand, if I had lupus, I was already doing many of the right things, thanks to my hypoglycemia—avoiding stress, eating well-balanced meals, and following a conservative lifestyle (no drinking or smoking).

I checked out several books about lupus, but before finishing any of them, I received the results of the second series of blood tests.

CHAPTER 8

"IT COULD BE CANCER"

After completing my pelvic exam. Dr. Lance reported, "You also have large fibroids in the uterus and perhaps endometriosis. The latter two are probably benign conditions." I was glad to hear that *something* might be benign. "An immediate hysterectomy may be necessary," he continued. "At your age, we recommend a complete hysterectomy."

"No," I found myself automatically responding. "I can't have surgery *now*." I began listing my reasons, including the wedding of my oldest niece.

"When is the wedding?" he asked gently.

"The Fourth of July weekend."

"You should be fairly well recovered by then," he assured me. "I don't see any problem with that."

I rattled off the rest of my excuses.

"If it's cancer," he interrupted, confronting the problem directly, "you don't want to wait."

Suddenly the urgency of this appointment shattered my illusions that cancer was not a concern. After months of impatience and uncertainty, a potential cause was revealed. Unexpectedly, events now were moving fast—too fast.

The day before, when Dr. Fields gave me the tentative diagnosis of lupus, I had dismissed the possibility of cancer, *preferring* the lupus diagnosis. Now, cancer loomed large in my present and future—a most foreboding presence.

"With ovarian masses," Dr. Lance said, interrupting my thoughts, "we can't be certain they aren't cancer until we go in surgically."

"But if it is cancer," I replied, frightened, "by now it's probably spread throughout my entire body. I've had this pain for ten years or more. It's only gotten worse in the last two years. Are you sure it's not just a cyst? My younger sister had an ovarian cyst removed a few years ago. Hers wasn't cancer. She had endometriosis too."

"I'd like to do an ultrasound test first," he explained. "That might give us a better idea of what we're dealing with and whether immediate surgery is needed."

"If it's cancer, I won't have surgery unless you can convince me it hasn't spread," I said, trying to set my own terms. I did not want my body cut open, only to have the doctors say they couldn't do anything because it had spread too extensively.

Dr. Lance scheduled the ultrasound test for the next day.

This can't be happening to me, I thought, feeling numb as I left the doctor's office. But I knew, all too painfully, that it was.

I called Bud at work and broke the news to him. Then I called my sister-in-law, Van, Bud's brother's wife and told her it looked like we would not be able to host the fiftieth anniversary celebration for Bud and Tom's parents. She accepted the news with more grace than I expected, since the bulk of the preparation would now fall on her shoulders.

My diary entries at this time convey the depth of my feelings:

Wednesday, March 24, 1982

I don't want to deal with the reality of hospitalization and especially with having my body cut into—this body that has never even been in a hospital, this body that I've taken such good care of all these years so I wouldn't have to undergo surgery, ever. I just can't believe I have cancer. I'm just starting to feel good again after being off the iron and vitamins for five months. Yesterday my blood count was 13.4, higher than it's been in eight years. And I've gained two pounds. That's not indicative of a body "wasting away" with cancer. I *won't* believe it. I *can't* believe I have *cancer*.

Bud and I went out to eat that night. I was in no mood to cook. On the way to the restaurant, we stopped at the neighborhood branch library. I checked out two books about hysterectomy and three about cancer. Before going to bed that night, I skimmed both hysterectomy books. None of the cancer books discussed ovarian cancer.

In my case, the only real indication of cancer was pain and anemia. But I had taken estrogen for more than a year; I believed that might increase my chances of having ovarian cancer. I decided I would have to do a lot of praying and trusting. The stress of uncertainty and decision-making would not help a lupus condition either.

Thursday, March 25, 1982
Last night I went to bed thinking I would *not* risk surgery *at any price*, but this morning, after much prayer, I feel differently. I am willing to discuss my options with Dr. Lance when the results of the ultrasound test come back.

In Marian Ropes's book, *Systemic Lupus Erythematosus*,[5] she claims surgery accelerates lupus in approximately one-third of patients. At this point, I still leaned heavily toward avoiding surgery because of the lupus risks—infection and pulmonary problems. Breathing difficulties still plagued me.

The big question remained: should I undergo surgery to rid my body of cancer and risk dying from complications of lupus, or should I reject the cancer surgery to extend my life with lupus? It was a no-win situation.

In the hour before the ultrasound test, I had to drink a half gallon

---

[5] Marian W. Ropes, MD. *Systemic Lupus Erythematosus* (Cambridge, MA, Harvard University Press, 1976).

of water. I thought a good pace would be one sixteen-ounce glassful every fifteen minutes. The first sixteen ounces went down easily. *Will my bladder be able to hold it all before the test?* I wondered. I drank the last sixteen ounces in the ultrasound waiting room, just as my hour expired. Actually, drinking a half gallon of water in an hour was not the ordeal I had expected. In fact, I hardly felt uncomfortable as I walked into the test room, located next door to the waiting room. *My bladder must be bigger than I thought*, I speculated. But I was glad to see a restroom nearby.

If I ever have to retake this test, I will make one minor change—I will *not* drink *ice* water. Half a gallon of ice water chills the body amazingly fast. I couldn't stop shivering during the entire procedure.

The technician smeared a jellylike substance on my bare abdomen. Then she moved a scanning head, which resembled a microphone, over the area to be diagnosed.

Ultrasound uses high-frequency sound waves to create a picture of the body's internal organs. Using a special camera technique, an image is reproduced, and photographs can be retained for diagnostic purposes. The pictures were flashed onto a monitoring screen that looked like a small black-and-white television set, located just above my head and off to one side. I watched the pictures appear and dissolve into one another as the scanning head moved, but of course I had no idea of what I was seeing. The heavy black spots, I suspected, were the trouble spots. Fortunately, I didn't see many of them.

With the test completed, the technician said, "You can let out a cup of urine if you feel uncomfortable." The pictures were checked to see if more were needed. I chose to stay put. I had no discomfort yet. "If I let out a cupful," I said, "I'll probably empty my whole bladder." I could not always stop the flow of urine once it started.

The technician took the pictures down to Dr. Lance's office. Upon her return, she announced, "He said they looked good." She further reassured me they would be read by another expert, who would report his findings to Dr. Lance. I emptied my bladder and went home.

I mistakenly took Dr. Lance's comment about them "looking good" to mean immediate surgery was not necessary. With lifted spirits, I left the ultrasound office. Still, I waited anxiously by the telephone for the next two days until the important call came.

At three o'clock on Friday afternoon, Dr. Lance called. The news was not good. He recommended surgery as soon as possible. The ultrasound test showed hard and soft spots in the mass. A cyst would only have soft spots.

"If it's cancer, can you tell if it has spread?" I asked anxiously.

"I want to run a kidney test first," he said. Then he added, as if it was an afterthought, "We can run a liver scan too. The kidney test will check the location of the organs. We don't want to accidentally cut the wrong thing." He laughed.

I recognized the comment as an attempt at levity to lighten the seriousness of our conversation, but I didn't feel lighthearted. "I certainly don't want you to cut the wrong thing either," I replied, solemnly agreeing to the tests he recommended.

"Which hospital would you like to go to for your surgery?" he asked.

"I haven't agreed to *have* surgery yet," I reminded him.

"I'm going to go ahead and schedule an operating room anyway." He spoke with authority. "Time is of the essence, and it's not always easy to get an operating room on short notice." As if to placate me, he added, "We can always cancel."

I gave him the name of my hospital of choice—Mercy General, our neighborhood hospital and close to his office; it had a good reputation.

"The nurse will give you the dates for your liver and kidneys scans," he said. One of the office girls came on the line with the information.

That was quick! I thought.

After hanging up, I called several women friends who I knew who had had hysterectomies. "Did you have to have liver or kidney scans before your surgery?" I inquired. No one did. But then, none of them had been diagnosed with cancer either.

Dr. Lance didn't say why he'd ordered the liver scan. I suspected it was to check for the spread of cancer. Later, I learned iron overdose can also damage the liver.

Next, I called Dr. Fields's office and asked for the results of the last two lupus tests. Both were negative, or normal—no indication of lupus. I was almost sorry to hear the news. Now, how could I excuse the bone pain? The respiratory problems? The swollen glands?

Even though the lupus tests were normal, I questioned whether I was free of the disease. From my research, I knew that when lupus goes into remission, it will not give a positive blood test result—it's as if the condition never existed. My last sedimentation rate of twenty-three, near normal, indicated I could be in a remission stage.

Still, I had read enough about lupus to know it was not a disease I desired. It could be as life-threatening as cancer. For the time being, I decided to put thoughts of lupus aside. I had other—more important—concerns to occupy my mind.

That night when a church member called with the weekly prayer chain, I asked to have my name added to the list. I needed all the prayer support I could get.

The next day, Saturday, I busied myself with housecleaning, trying to forget the liver and kidney tests scheduled for the following Tuesday—and the impending doom they represented. I looked forward to the noontime mail delivery, hoping it would bring news items for the next *Communicator* newsletter. I coveted the distraction of a creative work project to keep my mind off myself and my fears. But nothing came.

That night, I decided it was time for Bud and me to discuss the proposed surgery.

CHAPTER 9

"THREE YEARS TO LIVE"

"We need to talk about your surgery," Bud said, after supper on Saturday, March 27, broaching the subject we'd both sidestepped for days, beating me to my resolve to bring it up first. In my anxiety, I had discussed it with anyone who would listen to me, except Bud. Talking about it dispelled my fears, and helped me to accept facts I would have preferred to ignore. But Bud and I had not talked about it, as if by avoiding the discussion, we could avoid the surgery.

"Frankly," Bud began, sounding a little testy, "I'm a little jealous that you've talked to everyone else about your surgery but not to me."

I seethed, "I didn't think you wanted to talk about it. I didn't think you wanted to admit I had a problem—a serious problem. Whenever I mentioned my trips to the hematologist, you always seemed uninterested, as if you didn't care what I had to report. You never asked questions—"

"I am interested," Bud interrupted, "and I do care. I just don't believe in borrowing trouble."

"Well, I'm the type of person who needs to know everything," I explained. "I need to prepare myself. I need to decide what course of action to take before the action needs to be taken. Today I made a list of reasons for having the surgery and a list of reasons for not having the surgery. There are only two reasons for it but thirteen reasons *against* it." I had made up my mind. I didn't plan to have surgery. I held up the yellow legal pad so he could see my list.

Against Surgery

1. No excessive gushing or bleeding
2. Out of 750,000 hysterectomies annually, 12,000 women still die
3. Surgical complications from blood clots
4. Complications from diabetes
5. No current between-period bleeding
6. My periods are not irregular
7. Complications from lupus, if I have lupus in remission
8. No history of ovarian cancer in my family
9. Possible weight loss from surgery [I didn't want to lose more weight.]
10. Estrogen replacement therapy following surgery; its effect on my cystic breasts
11. My last pap test was normal
12. Pulmonary complications with surgery [I still experienced breathing difficulties.]
13. Lupus; possible risk of kidney problems

And I hadn't even mentioned that it could destroy our sex life. I knew he'd care about *that*.

The list "For Surgery" looked inconsequential in comparison, but the two items carried a great deal of weight.

For Surgery

1. Pain
2. Cancer

"I don't *want* to have surgery," I wailed, as the tears started to fall. I felt trapped in a no-win situation.

"If it means saving your life, baby, you've got to have the surgery," Bud said gently.

"I don't *have* to have it!" I exploded, frustrated by the lack of choices but not really angry at him. "And if it *is* cancer and it has spread, I'm not going to have it. I won't have them going in and spreading it throughout my whole body." I paused for a minute to catch my breath between sobs. "I guess what it really boils down to is this: I just don't want anyone cutting into my body." I finally admitted this vanity, both to myself and to him. "I've never even been in a hospital, except to visit. Forty-three years old, and I thought I was in perfect health. I don't smoke. I eat properly. I seldom drink alcohol. I visit my doctor every year and have my yearly pelvic and pap exams. I've tried to keep my body healthy so I wouldn't have to have surgery—not ever. It's not fair."

My holistic doctors had totally convinced me that by "living right," I could prevent illness. Now, I found it all to be a lie. How do you prevent cancer—or even ovarian cysts?

"I want my body to remain virgin. I don't want anyone cutting into it." A flood of fresh tears rushed over me.

"Your body is no longer *virgin*," Bud murmured with a smile.

But I rebuffed his attempt at levity. "That's not what I meant, and you know it," I snapped.

Of course he knew exactly what I meant, and he listened patiently as I raged on, hugging me when he thought it appropriate, holding me close when my body was wracked with sobs as I stubbornly fought the battle with myself, trying to rationalize a way out of having surgery. He made appropriate comments when he found the opportunity to do so, but mostly he just listened.

"I suppose I should tell you this too," I said, gulping between sobs.

He stared at me, curious about a new revelation, but he did not speak.

"Last year I had a premonition," I began. "I don't remember exactly when it came to me—early in the summer, I think; maybe June—that I only had three years left to live, that I only had three years in which to do all the things I thought I needed to do before I died. You know my premonitions often come true."

He nodded. His expression remained grave and concerned.

"I've already used up almost a whole year," I said through my tears. "There are things I want to do before I die—articles I want to write. If I only have two years left, I don't want to waste even a part of them recuperating from an operation. I don't want to lose even six weeks when I can be doing other things. I'd rather not have the operation than to lose some of the valuable time I have left."

"I want you to have the surgery," he said firmly, "because I want you to live. I want you to spend the rest of your life with me. And if you only have two years left ... well, we'll deal with that too. But let's not borrow trouble. Don't assume you have cancer until the doctor tells you that you do. I just want you to know that I want you to have this surgery. I won't think you are less a woman because of it—"

"*I* am the one who has to want the surgery," I interrupted, flinging the words at him. "It's *my life*, not yours. It's *my body* that's being cut into. It's my life that's on the line. It has to be *my* decision—not yours. *I* have to decide." It was a responsibility that, at the moment, I wished I could relinquish, but I knew I could not.

"That's true," Bud agreed calmly. "In the final analysis, *you* have to make the decision because it is your life. I just wanted you to understand how I feel. I want you to live. And if this operation will help you live longer, I want you to have it. And if it's cancer, we'll deal with that if we have to."

"You don't even know the risks of surgery," I snapped. "It's easy for you to say, 'Have surgery.' Thousands of women still die on the operating table—or afterwards—from complications. What if I die in surgery? Before you are so quick to convince me to have surgery, maybe you'd better read up on the complications." I flung the book I was reading at him, citing the chapter that dealt with the complications of hysterectomy. It landed on the lamp table that separated our two easy chairs.

He didn't open it or even reach for it. I didn't expect him to. He didn't want to know the worst.

"And what if I'm not *supposed* to have this operation?" I challenged.

"What if God doesn't want me to have surgery, and I go ahead anyway, on my own, and die on the operating table because I didn't trust Him enough? Then I won't have even two years left."

For almost a year I had lived with my secret fear that my life was ending. It was a relief, finally, to acknowledge it and share the burden with someone else—to voice it so it could be examined objectively and rationally analyzed. Holistic medicine had done a number on me with their brainwashing techniques. I was convinced that if I trusted God completely, He would heal me without human intervention. This was a gross distortion of God's healing principle. God gives His gifts of healing to people—some are doctors—who can use their gifts for good or evil. Unfortunately, some medical professionals use their knowledge to make and keep their patients sick. People become profitable long-term care patients.

Emotionally spent, I reviewed what holistic medicine had taught me: God wants you to be a healthy, whole person in control of your own life and health. That was a lie! God, not I, was in control. I had never been in control; I only had a false delusion of power.

Finally, I had cried out all the anger, rage, and frustration over this situation in which I had no control. In the past, I'd prided myself on not being a sentimental person, not one easily reduced to tears, but these tears were helpful. A good cry, I'd heard, cleanses the soul.

Bud's outward expression remained calm and concerned throughout my temperamental outburst. When I finally finished raging, he gathered me in his arms, held me close, and said, "The premonition came before you changed doctors. Maybe it was only meant to be a warning—a warning that if you *didn't* have this surgery, you would only have three years to live. If you hadn't changed doctors, you still might not know you even *needed* surgery. If it should be malignant, and you only have two more years to live, we'll deal with it—together. I'll always be here because I love you. But don't assume you have cancer until the doctor tells you so."

"I'm not *assuming* I have cancer," I stormed again, frustrated because he still did not understand my motivation. "I'm *preparing* myself for that eventuality. Can't you understand? If it is cancer, I need to make certain decisions—in advance. I need to know what the next course of action is going to be *before* the verdict comes in. Don't think for a moment I'm giving up hope. I want to live just as much as you want me to. But we have to discuss death; it is a possibility, you know."

Death—that was the real subject, the one we didn't want to confront. Death and loss and all the gloomy feelings that come with the end of life.

We discussed funeral arrangements. I knew Bud would have preferred to skip that discussion, but I had certain requests about my funeral service that he needed to know.

That night, I realized that Bud and I viewed life from two different philosophical perspectives. Bud, in not wanting to "borrow trouble," avoided problems until they absolutely, of necessity, had to be confronted. I considered this an "ostrich with its head in the sand" approach. One cannot make valid decisions with incomplete information or information obtained at the eleventh hour under duress. Under those circumstances, a person simply does not have time to accumulate the necessary facts and data to make sound, informed judgments.

I, on the other hand, needed to see the whole picture—the good, the bad, and the ugly. I needed to weigh good and bad alternatives equally, examining all options in order to understand why some procedures are favored over others. I preferred to be prepared for the worst and have it *not* come to pass than to be filled with false hope and have it dashed by reality. Serious problems cannot be wished away, nor can they be avoided by ignoring them. One must be fully informed in order to make the right choices.

This is where holistic medicine fails. It refuses to confront illness or negative health issues, preferring to concentrate only on the positive aspects of health.

Later, as I mulled over what Bud had said, I wondered if he could be right. Perhaps the premonition was given to me as a warning that I needed to find a new doctor—one with expert medical knowledge, one I could trust to tell me the truth about my medical condition, one who could save my life. I hadn't thought about it that way before. Maybe Bud spoke the truth. I knew he spoke with love. I clutched at that straw of hope. We never know when God is going to speak to us through the voice of another person.

I looked at Bud in a new light that night. For the first time I saw a spiritual strength and understanding I didn't know he possessed. And in that revelation, new love and respect blossomed.

CHAPTER 10

TESTS AND QUESTIONS

As we walked into church on Sunday morning, March 28, Carl and Harriet Hammon, our elderly neighborhood friends, greeted us with bear hugs. I seemed to need more hugs these days. Their hugs provided an extra measure of strength and comfort. Bud also was more demonstrative of late. Perhaps he too needed the strength and comfort that comes from hugging and having someone share your burden.

I kept telling myself, *I feel too good—too healthy—to have cancer.* Then I'd get a twinge of pain in my abdomen or a stitch in my chest while taking a deep breath, and I'd remember that cancer can be a silent killer.

I needed to tuck in many loose ends before surgery. On Monday, March 29, I stopped at Dr. Lance's office to sign the medical release forms, enabling them to get my records from Dr. Fields.

From there, I went to a diagnostic lab in the building for more blood tests—a presurgical SMAC (Chem 20) test to check electrolyte balances in the blood (calcium, sodium, potassium, etc.) – twenty different blood tests, including one for blood sugar. Before noon, I had to pick up the IVP (intravenous pyelogram) kit for the kidney scan. The kit contained diet information and a laxative to empty the bowels before the scan. Nine years ago, Bud had had the same kidney test. I couldn't remember anything about it, except that it was painless.

Monday, March 29, 1982

I am actually starting to look forward to surgery as an end to this uncertainty. If it is cancer, I now feel surgery will show there has been no spread. The longer surgery is delayed, the more time prayer has to work—hopefully to reverse and heal the condition. I feel like everyone in the world is praying for me; I'm very much at peace, regardless of what Bud thinks.

Bud gets irritated with what he terms my "negative attitude." But he cannot feel the body pain, the bone aches, the breathing tightness, or throbbing lymph glands. It's easy to be optimistic when you don't hurt. I think I'm being quite positive about the negative aspects of my condition.

At noon I started the IVP diet. It required me to eat more than I usually eat for lunch—bouillon soup with crackers, turkey sandwich (white meat; no butter, mayonnaise, or lettuce), apple juice, skim milk, and gelatin. I also had to drink measured amounts of water at specified times.

Monday, March 29, 1982 (later)

This afternoon I finished six pages of the district newsletter—only two more pages to go. I am so thankful to have this creative mental diversion to keep my mind off the tests scheduled for tomorrow.

I didn't think I was anxious about the tests, but at eight o'clock that night, I realized I had forgotten to feed Mitzi, our little black cockapoo. Three hours late. No wonder she'd been following me around the house, grunting.

By evening I was hungry, too, and especially thirsty. Normally, I drank most of my daily intake of water in the evening, but according to instructions, I could only eat and drink at the times specified and only the amounts and types of food specified.

That night, I noticed I could take deep breaths—without pain. Had the healing process already begun? Was God healing me?

For the liver scan, a technician injected radioactive iodine into my arm. After a ten-minute wait for the body to absorb the material, she took the x-rays while I was fully clothed. Had I known I would not have to undress, I would not have worn a western shirt with metal buttons. The blouse had to be opened and all the metal buttons tucked underneath my body away from the x-ray plates.

"We don't want to have some unexplained little dots on your liver," the technician explained. I asked about the test, and she said it scanned the liver and spleen but not the lungs.

For the IVP kidney test, I disrobed, removed all metal, and put on a heavy hospital gown. After a few preliminary x-rays, the technician asked whether I was allergic to iodine or seafood.

"No, I love lobster," I replied.

A doctor came in and started the radioactive iodine IV drip. The iodine made my body feel warm all over. In the cool x-ray room, the hot flush of the intravenous solution felt almost pleasant. The doctor warned that the IV might cause shortness of breath or itching and advised that I should notify him immediately if either occurred. I experienced no such reactions.

Halfway through the procedure, I noticed I still was wearing my metal penicillin-allergy necklace. Fearing that the metal in the necklace might interfere with the kidney x-rays, I mentioned it to the technician.

"If your kidneys are *that high*," he replied, trying to suppress a chuckle, "you've really got a problem." We both laughed.

I lost track of the number of x-rays taken—many more than for the liver scan. When the test ended, the technician said, "Your doctor will have the results tomorrow morning."

With the testing over, I felt slightly depressed. I called Bud at work and then drove to visit my friend Helen. I needed to be with *people*. Her sister, who I knew from college days, was visiting from Wisconsin. It was a pleasant, relaxing few hours of diversion; we talked about many things, including my impending surgery. I was home by three o'clock.

Shortly thereafter, the call came from Dr. Lance's office. "Your surgery is scheduled for Monday, April 12, at seven-thirty in the morning." I would be admitted on April 11—Easter Sunday. "Your presurgery conference is scheduled with Dr. Lance on Friday, April 9, at 4:15 p.m."

"I have to talk to him *before* that date," I said. "I have too many questions that need to be resolved before I consent to surgery. If they are not resolved, there will be no surgery. I have not given my consent to have surgery."

She rescheduled my appointment for April 1.

Tuesday, March 30, 1982

Bud is still concerned about what he calls my "fatalistic attitude." For months, I've been reading voraciously on a variety of subjects: anemia, hematology, inspirational books, the psychology of positive thinking, and now, hysterectomy, cancer, and lupus—whatever I can find in the library pertaining to my condition. To my dismay, our library is sadly deficient in information about ovarian cancer—either in book form or magazine articles. I've read so much medical jargon, I'm starting to understand it.

Bud is afraid my reading program, which is designed to prepare me for the worst, will cause me to lose hope and stop fighting to live if I become convinced the problem *is* cancer. He doesn't understand that even if the doctors say my case is hopeless, I will still have hope. I have experienced God in action. How can I convince my husband that you can't deal with a problem until you've *identified* it?

I've read some excellent inspirational books in order to put myself in the proper frame of mind for this surgery. Dr. Arnold A. Hutschnecker's *The Will to Live*[6] was especially helpful. He points out that people tend to react in one of two ways when confronted with a crisis: fight or flight. Bud, I think, tends toward flight, whereas I, I decided, am a fighter.

---

[6] Arnold A. Hutschnecker, MD. *The Will to Live* (Prentice Hall, Inc.: Englewood, NJ, 1951, 1958).

Late Wednesday afternoon, March 31, I called Dr. Fields's office and asked to speak to him. "My presurgery conference with Dr. Lance is scheduled for tomorrow," I told him. "Before I decide to have surgery, I need answers to some questions."

"Okay," he said.

"In your expert opinion, why do you think I'm anemic?"

"I don't really know," he replied. "Your test results show that, for some reason, you seem to have hypoproliferative bone marrow [produces less red blood cells than normal], which now seems to be acting normally. Your last hemoglobin count was 13.4."

"Do you think the excessive iron caused the anemia?"

"No," he answered, "but it might have caused the high sedimentation rate, which is now almost back to normal. Your last sed rate was twenty-three."

"Do any of the blood tests you've taken indicate I have cancer?"

"No, not in my opinion," he replied, "but one cannot always tell by blood tests. Blood tests can be normal, and cancer can still be present. Ovarian cancer is especially hard to detect until surgery is performed. And until then, we can't always tell if it has spread."

I was relieved to hear him reaffirm what Dr. Lance, my gynecologist, had already said, and it gave me renewed confidence in my doctors.

"And I don't have lupus?"

"The first lupus test showed only a slight abnormality, more like a low normal. The second ANA and C-3 tests were both normal. You have a lot of strange and unexplained symptoms," he said.

"The protein electrophoresis test you did was for bone cancer, wasn't it?"

"Myeloma."

"Isn't that bone cancer?"

"It's one type of bone cancer; there are different kinds of bone cancer."

"But it was okay, wasn't it?"

"It was normal."

"In your opinion, is there any reason I should *not* have this surgery?"

"No. Your hemoglobin count is within a normal range now. Your sedimentation rate is almost normal. If you need the surgery, you should have it." He asked when the surgery was scheduled, and I gave him the date. "Keep me posted about the results," he said.

Impressed with his genuine concern, I added his name to the list of people I wanted Bud to call with the surgery results.

By mid-afternoon, curious about the results of the liver and kidney scans, I called Dr. Lance's office.

"They aren't in yet," the receptionist said, "but we'll make sure we have them by your appointment tomorrow afternoon."

Patience, I thought. *I must learn patience.*

Thursday finally arrived. The *big day*. The day I'd get the test results. The day I had to make my final decision about surgery, although now it seemed inevitable. After much research, I concluded that if it *was* cancer, even if it had spread, surgery *was* necessary. First, you remove the primary cancer; then you treat the secondary cancer(s).

I typed a whole page of questions, single-spaced, to ask Dr. Lance the next day.

CHAPTER 11

THE DECISION IS MADE

"Your liver test was normal," Dr. Lance said, holding up the written report so we could see the word NORMAL typed on the paper. It gave me a renewed sense of confidence. He was sharing all pertinent information with Bud and me.

"Just why did you order the liver scan?" I asked. "None of my friends had liver scans."

"If ovarian cancer spreads, it usually invades the liver first," he said, verifying my suspicions. "The kidney test shows a mass has already begun to deviate the left ureter [the tube that runs from the kidney to the bladder], pushing it out of alignment but not yet enough to interfere with urine flow. This is the type of information I need. Not knowing that it had moved from where it is supposed to be, I accidentally might have cut the wrong thing. The kidney test also does not indicate cancer involvement."

I found that reassuring, but he was quick to point out, "We do not really know for sure if cancer is present until we visually examine the tissue around the organ and test the mass for malignancy. When the mass is removed, it will be quick-frozen. Some thin tissue slices will be removed. The pathologist will inspect them under a microscope immediately. If malignant cells are found, the surgeons will give the surrounding tissue closer inspection, checking for cancer spread. In that case, I might have to go as high as the liver with the visual inspection; otherwise, I won't disturb that part of your body.

"Even if the frozen section is benign, they will continue to check sections of the tumor from different areas, in case the first section just happened to be from a benign area. The initial tissue report is correct 90 percent of the time, but a complete subsectioning of the tumor takes about three days. It is checked quite thoroughly to make sure no cancer cells are overlooked."

"What if you find a malignancy after the three days of checking? Do you reopen me to remove it?"

"There are other ways to treat ovarian cancer. We'll discuss that later if we *have* to."

"What did my last pap smear show?"

"Your last pap test was normal," he said, "as was the estrogen level for your age."

I mentally noted that in December I'd discontinued the estrogen Betty had prescribed. *Did I ever need it?*

"Will I have to take estrogen *after* surgery?" I asked.

"Unless I find cancer, I'll probably put you on estrogen therapy for five years after surgery."

"But I have cystic breasts. Won't estrogen make that condition worse? I've heard it can lead to breast cancer."

"In recent studies, estrogen has been found *not* to accelerate breast cancer," he replied. "From the studies now, it seems, certain women are just more predisposed to breast cancer than others. Taking or not taking estrogen seems to have no correlation to acquiring breast cancer. Mostly, estrogen is found to accelerate cancers of the uterus and sometimes the ovaries, but progesterone seems to have a retarding effect on some ovarian cancers."

"Can you tell me if the ovarian mass is on the inside or outside of the ovary?"

"The ultrasound shows the mass to be *inside* the ovary."

At least it appeared to be contained. I breathed a sigh of relief.

"We have to operate on the assumption the mass is cancerous," he explained. "When we are unsure, we must assume it *is* cancer because it makes a difference in how we do our cutting. We don't want to spread cancer cells."

"Are ovarian tumors usually painful?"

"Ovarian tumors that are cancerous do not cause pain all the time. There is no definite pattern."

"You said the ultrasound showed hard *and* soft masses. Aren't cancerous tumors usually hard?"

"Cancerous tumors are usually hard, but not all hard tumors are cancerous."

"Can ovarian cancer spread to the bone?"

"Ovarian cancers usually only spread to the bone in very late stages of the disease," he answered. "Seldom does the process work in reverse—from bone cancer to ovarian."

"Is there any alternative to surgery?" I asked. "Can't you biopsy beforehand to see if surgery is necessary?"

"There is no alternative treatment to surgery," he patiently replied. "Until we actually see the organs, we cannot make an accurate diagnosis. There is no way to biopsy for ovarian cancer." (After surgery, I understood why it was unwise to biopsy.)

"I think I've had this tumor—or whatever it is—for at least ten years or more without major problems. Is that a good indication it may *not* be cancer?"

"I cannot assure you of that."

"If it has spread to nearby organs—to the kidney or spleen—will you remove those organs during surgery?"

"No," he assured me, "those are major, vital organs. We have other methods of treatment."

"If it is cancerous, what follow-up treatments will I have to undergo?"

He refused to discuss postoperative treatments for cancer with us. "There are many different kinds of ovarian cancer," he said. "The treatment is a little different for each type. If necessary, we will discuss that aspect after surgery."

I didn't blame him for not wanting to discuss all the ramifications of cancer treatment, especially if it turned out to be unnecessary. He took the same non-discussion stance toward proposed treatments, should the cancer have spread to other organs. The treatment depended on where the cancer had spread and whether the spread was new or advanced. He would discuss it only if necessary.

"Will I need a blood transfusion?" I asked, wondering if I needed to bank some of my blood for the surgery.

"With a hysterectomy, there is minimal need for blood transfusions, but I always cross-type and have a few pints available, in case it is needed."

"Will I be able to eat Easter dinner?" *What kind of Easter dinner would I get,* I wondered, *would the hospital serve a traditional Easter meal?*

"You can eat normally the day before surgery, but all water and food will be taken away after midnight. You will be on an intravenous solution, and you probably will not eat for two or three days after surgery."

"How will I take my thyroid medication? My holistic doctor warned not to skip any doses."

"Normally, you shouldn't. You can take your next day's dosage before midnight on the night before surgery. It won't cause any major problems to be without it for two or three days, until you can take fluids and food orally. You will be pretty doped up the first day. I urge you to take all your pain shots the first day. They don't give out hero badges for enduring pain." I skipped from subject to subject on my list.

"After seven hours without food, I get hypoglycemic. How will you prevent shock?"

"The dextrose intravenous feedings will take care of that. Your surgery is scheduled for 7:30 in the morning. I probably will not actually start surgery until closer to eight." He turned to Bud. "If you want to see her before surgery, you'd better plan to be at the hospital about six." Bud nodded agreement.

Returning the conversation to me, he said, "Before you leave your hospital room, you'll be given a heavy dose of sodium pentothal—truth serum. It will probably knock you out cold, so you won't spill all the family secrets, as sometimes happens when a mild dose is given. If all goes well, you should be out of surgery by ten o'clock. As soon as the tumor is removed, it will be quick-frozen, sliced, stained, and checked for malignant cells. If no malignancy is found, we will continue with the surgery and close."

"Will I have a bikini incision?" I wanted a small incision.

"Your incision will probably run from the pelvic bone to the belly button. If we have to check the liver, it could run from the pelvic bone to the breast bone."

"Do you remove the appendix at the same time?"

"I do not remove the appendix as a matter of course. If it is not readily accessible and looks healthy, I'll probably leave it alone. If it is readily accessible and removal looks simple, I may remove it."

"How long will I be hospitalized?"

"The usual hospital stay is one week; it could be longer if there are complications." He would not discuss when I could start doing things again after surgery. "It depends on the severity of the surgery. We'll discuss that just before I release you to go home."

"I am now agreeable to having the surgery," I told him, "or at least I'm resigned to the idea. I know it has to be done." As we shook hands, preparatory to our leaving, I said to him with all sincerity, "I have every confidence that you will do a good job."

Bud told Dr. Lance he was impressed with the doctor's professional attitude, his manner, and his knowledge. I added my agreement. Dr. Lance returned the compliment, saying he was impressed that we had our questions organized and written down and also by the fact I had extensively researched the subject and had talked with friends who had had hysterectomies.

The one thing I hadn't understood was his explanation of the "calcium deposits" in my abdomen that were discovered on the x-ray taken at the hospital in December. My concern was whether these deposits would complicate surgery. He said the deposits had something to do with my body's not utilizing calcium properly. I made a mental note to ask for further clarification when he came to visit me in the hospital on Sunday night to answer last-minute questions. A new list of questions was already formulating in my mind.

As we walked to the car, Bud commented, "He looks so *young*."

"He'll have steady hands," I replied. I wanted a nice, straight incision, not a jagged scar. *Vanity, vanity, thy name is woman,* flashed into my mind.

I had checked the medical diplomas hanging on the wall in his office. He had at least six years of experience as a surgeon. I was confident that was enough.

In spite of all my questions, the meeting lasted only half an hour. The decision was made; I would have the surgery. Relief flooded over me, as if a heavy burden had been lifted.

CHAPTER 12

TWO FRIENDS: THE OLD

I believe that God puts certain people in our lives at certain times for certain reasons. Sometimes we don't understand the reasons until years or even decades later.

For twenty years, I'd wondered about my friend Debbie. Since leaving the Midwest to move to Arizona, I tried sporadically to locate her—a futile effort. I didn't hold much hope of ever seeing her again. We'd lost touch even before I left Minneapolis. If she'd searched for me, it was unlikely she'd have thought to look out West. So I searched for her, but not diligently; I had little hope of success. She'd probably moved as far away from our hometown as I had. Our chances of reconnecting were slim.

Debbie and I met on the school bus during my last year of high school. High school was not a particularly happy period in my life; I was an intelligent farm girl in a small town, where no one valued "brainy" kids. Today I might be classified a lonely nerd. I was one of only five girls in my senior class. My leisure time and finances were limited, so I had to forgo congregating with classmates after school at the local hamburger hangout, where close personal friendships developed. At the end of the school day, I had to catch the rural school bus for a monotonous hour-long ride home. Although my parents lived only three miles from the school, the bus route ran backward. My brothers and I boarded last in the morning but were dropped off last at night.

Debbie, a seventh grader new to the community that year, seemed shy and reserved, yet warm and sensitive; she was an unusually mature and intelligent girl for her age. I remembered her as a happy child, a fellow Christian. We worshipped in the same church denomination but did not attend the same church.

Debbie lived toward the middle of the bus route. We enjoyed visiting with each other after friends in our own age groups had been dropped off. Conversation helped dispel the tedium of an otherwise dreary daily bus ride. As the weeks passed, I looked forward to our stimulating conversations. We talked about school, our families, current events, religion, and our hopes and dreams for the future. And I shared some of my early writings with Debbie.

Debbie seemed to enjoy our visits too. Perhaps she was flattered to have the high school senior-class president pay attention to her. I don't know if she viewed our association as giving her status or making her more acceptable among her peers. I didn't care. To me, being senior-class president wasn't anything special. I knew I had not been elected because of my popularity but because it was a job no one else wanted. It came with responsibilities and duties; arranging class reunions after graduation headed the list.

While Debbie and I were friendly, we both had other friends on the school bus and off. Our friendship, basically borne of loneliness and a desire to be accepted, was a special partnership that blossomed into a solid, warm kinship and continued through letters after I graduated high school and attended college.

When we did finally reconnect, after decades apart, it struck me as being preordained, arranged by a power greater than either of us could have imagined or understood.

My mother knew about my interest in renewing my friendship with Debbie. One day toward the end of our two-week visit, she said, "I hear Debbie Johnson is teaching in the Maple Plain school district." A year earlier, Mother had given me this same information. Dutifully, I checked it out with a college classmate who taught in the same district.

At Christmastime, my friend wrote, "No one in our school district ever heard of Debbie. Sorry."

"You probably have her confused with her sister, Beth," I told Mom after explaining the previous year's futile search.

"No, I'm sure it's Debbie," Mom insisted. "You can always check with her mother. I think she still works at the old grade school."

"If Bud and I have time tomorrow, maybe we'll stop," I answered, more to placate my mother's curiosity than my own. Bud and I planned to visit my country grade school teacher the next day. Mrs. Landry, retired now, lived close to the town grade school.

On past occasions when Bud and I had visited my parents in the summer, the public schools were closed—there had been no opportunity to learn about Debbie through her mother. After the death of Debbie's father, her mother had moved, but I never bothered to find out where. I rationalized that Debbie had made no effort to contact me through my parents, who still lived in the same house as when I was in high school. The reason for the demise of our friendship wasn't hard to diagnose: death by neglect.

It was September 1981. Bud and I had returned to Wisconsin for the wedding of my second niece, Carole. With schools in session, fate took a hand. I couldn't recall the name of the street where Mrs. Landry lived, nor could I recognize her house.

"Mrs. Johnson will probably know the address," I assured Bud as we pulled into the school parking lot. The two women were long-time school acquaintances.

When we arrived in Mrs. Johnson's office, she had just left for her coffee break. We waited.

Upon her return, I extended my hand in greeting. "Remember me?" I asked. She took my hand, warmly, but admitted she did not recognize me. I introduced myself, stating both my maiden and my married names. Then I introduced Bud.

"Of course, Debbie's friend." She smiled in recognition.

"What's Debbie doing now? I asked eagerly.

"She's teaching in Maple Plain."

Mother had been right. "And what's her name now?"

"Johnson. She's still single."

Now I was provoked that my college friend had failed to locate Debbie last year. I could have understood if Debbie had married and changed her last name. I wondered whether my friend actually had tried to locate her.

Mrs. Johnson and I chatted briefly about Debbie and her two siblings, who I also knew from the school bus ride. Finally, she gave us directions for finding Mrs. Landry's house. As we prepared to leave, Mrs. Johnson suggested, "Why don't you stop down at school and see Debbie. She'd love to see you again."

Love to? I wondered. Would she really love to see me again? I wasn't even sure I wanted to see her again. Would she love to have me pop in on her at work, unannounced? I wouldn't. I'm the type of person who doesn't like surprises. I prefer to have a degree of control over the circumstances in my life. Besides, I rationalized, when would we have time to stop to see her? Bud's and my remaining days of vacation were filled with family activities.

But cats and journalists share a common characteristic—we are innately curious creatures. I was a journalist and a writer. Remembering the premonition that I had only three years to live, I convinced myself, *This may be my last and only chance to see my old friend.*

Now I wondered: when did we stop corresponding? I couldn't remember. Losing a friend is like losing your eyesight. It's a gradual process—a slow erosion, marked by time, hardly noticeable until one day you wake up and realize—it's gone!

There were so many things I wanted to know about Debbie. Where had she gone to college? Does she like what she is doing? Has she remained the same sweet, sensitive person I remembered?

Fear had kept me from vigorously pursuing my search for Debbie. Fear that with the passage of time, she'd have changed and *wouldn't* be the same person. Fear that she might not wish to renew our friendship.

Fear that I might be regarded as an unwelcome intrusion from her past—an unhappy part of a lonely past that she might prefer to forget, as I sometimes did.

I remembered getting an announcement for Debbie's high school graduation. By then, I had graduated from college and was working for a publishing house in Minneapolis. As a graduation gift, I sent her a book. Now I couldn't recall if I ever received a thank-you note. Did Debbie stop writing first? Or did I? The question haunted me. Finally, I decided *she* must have stopped. As a writer, I wrote to everyone and anyone. Someone once told me that writers write, not because they have something to say, but because they have to say something. I wrote because I had to write.

Something within my body and my soul made me write. In writing, I perfected my craft—and I wanted to be perfect. Only then would I write seriously for publication. The cult of perfection—that earthly flaw that keeps so many people from achieving their potential.

In the early years following college graduation, I dreamed of writing the great, all-American novel. But as years passed, I realized I was not a novelist. Undaunted, I changed my aspirations, still determined to write and publish a book, perhaps several books, about life as it is really lived—if any writer can *ever* do that.

When faced with the prospect of death, friendships took on a new, special dimension for me—they became more important. It was important that I locate all the special people in my life (like my country grade school teacher), who had helped shape the person I had become, to let them know how much I appreciated their gift to me. I wanted to leave a legacy of love and gratitude.

So we asked directions to Debbie's school, located in an area unfamiliar to me. I expected Mrs. Johnson to write down the directions or at least draw a simple map. Lately, oral instructions and my brain did not mesh properly. Since my holistic treatment for iron deficiency anemia, I experienced more than the usual problems with assimilating verbal information. My mental capabilities could not absorb complicated directions, especially in an unfamiliar area. At times, my mind seemed to go numb—like computer circuits that automatically shut down when overloaded.

Unaware of my problem, Mrs. Johnson rattled off the directions as only one familiar with the area can do.

"I'll never remember that," I protested, but Bud said he could.

"Your brother took us by that new school once," he said. "Remember?"

I shook my head. What did it matter if I didn't remember as long as he could find it? He was driving.

"How late does Debbie stay at school?" I asked, "We're supposed to meet my brother and family for dinner tonight. Perhaps we can stop for a while beforehand."

"She's generally there until four o'clock, but she might leave early. We have stewardship dinners at church tonight."

At least she still attends church, I thought. We thanked Mrs. Johnson for the information and left to visit Mrs. Landry.

After lunch, Dad asked Bud to drive him into town. Mother and I rode along to visit my grandmother. By the time we returned home and dressed to meet my brother, Harold, and family for dinner, it was three-thirty. Maple Plain was a half-hour drive away.

Perhaps we're just not destined to meet again, I thought glumly. I was even more convinced when Bud couldn't find the street where Mrs. Johnson told him to turn. Complicating matters, neither of us remembered the name of the school.

"Let's just forget it," I suggested. "Maybe I can look her up another year." *I'll call first next time*, I thought. "We can go to Harold's and visit with Jimmy." My brother and Jean, his wife, both worked, but Jimmy, their twelve-year-old son would be home from school.

Bud refused to be deterred. "It should be right around here someplace," he insisted, finally stopping to ask directions from a pedestrian. "Can you tell us if there is a grade school nearby?"

The walker directed us to a school a few blocks away.

At exactly four o'clock, we drove into the school parking lot.

The school name, printed in large block letters on the building, still was unfamiliar.

"You go in and see if you can find her," Bud urged, "I'll wait here."

I walked into the school office, thankful that from my substitute teacher experience, I knew where to begin my search. "Does Debbie Johnson work here?" I asked the school secretary.

She confirmed that Debbie did work there and had not yet left for the day. She then gave directions for finding her, promising, "You can't miss her."

If you know what she looks like, I thought. After twenty years, I doubted I would recognize her, even if I did see her.

I didn't see her. *Should I just leave and forget the whole idea? Maybe this is God's way of telling me to let the past bury its dead.* I decided to tell Bud I couldn't find her; we had wasted the trip and our time.

Lost in this reverie, a maintenance man interrupted my thoughts. "Are you looking for someone," he asked.

"Debbie Johnson," I replied.

"She's in that meeting over there." He pointed to a group of teachers I had passed after entering a large open-area classroom. "I'll get her for you."

My view of the group was now obscured by six-foot-tall steel storage cabinets used to separate the teaching areas. The moment of truth had arrived—and I wanted to run, to quietly exit the building without seeing my friend. But I waited, rooted to the spot.

"My God," I pleaded silently. "What am I doing here? Did *you* send me for a reason?"

As if in answer to my breathed question, the story of the boy, Samuel, flashed into my mind, along with the command, *"Speak, Lord, for your servant hears."*

Here I am, Lord, I prayed silently. *Tell me what I'm doing here.* But no further messages came. I often spoke to God in this strange telepathic manner. As a child, I'd wished for the gift of prophecy—the ability to see into the future. But now, as an adult, when I caught what seemed to be glimpses of the future through strange and nebulous messages, like this one, they troubled me. I was not certain anymore that I wanted to be responsible for that kind of power or responsibility. Was premonition, or precognition, as some people called it, a blessing or a curse? Often the meanings were hidden and unclear for months— even years. What did this one mean?

Perfect love casts out fear. It was a fleeting response. I knew God would reveal the full meaning in His own time.

Just then, Debbie and the janitor appeared from behind the storage cabinets. She looked older and now taller than me. The round, childlike features in the face I remembered had thinned to angular, almost sharp proportions. Deep wrinkles etched her forehead. Her hair, cut in a short, easy-care style, showed gray hairs in front. Although five years my junior, she had more gray hair than I did. *Have I changed as much in appearance?* I wondered.

Her face, set in a grim, serious expression, sharpened the angular features into a glare. "Yes?" she said curtly, as if resenting this late-afternoon intrusion from a stranger.

"Remember me?" I asked, fastening a broad smile on my face. I wondered, if I'd been similarly challenged, would I have recognized her? *No*, I decided, *I certainly would not.*

"Of course I do." She smiled now, and the smile lighted her whole face. The smile had remained unchanged from early adolescence. It radiated and stripped years from her age—twenty years vanished in that smile. My lost friend had been found. My heart leaped with joy.

Impulsively, I stepped forward, wrapping my arms around her. "It's so good to see you again." The hug was brief and casual, but I sensed she had not anticipated it—perhaps had not even welcomed it. Her body stiffened momentarily, then relaxed slightly as she returned the quick embrace.

I guess she's not used to having people hug her, I thought. Still, her reaction disturbed me. We were, after all, old friends. Yet I empathized with her. Until a few years ago, open displays of physical affection were difficult for me too.

Then I'd attended a church women's convention. One of the themes that year was "Three hugs a day prevents skin hunger." We did a lot of hugging at that convention. My skin, I learned, was very hungry, so I set about correcting the deficiency. I found it easier now to hug people, especially when I was happy or if I hadn't seen the person for a long time.

But I realized that large numbers of people are not conditioned to open displays of physical affection. They are uncomfortable when such emotions are thrust upon them. How well I could relate to Debbie's discomfort. For years, I too suffered from it.

I stepped back quickly to look at her again.

"It's been a long time," she said simply.

"Must be twenty years," I agreed.

Over the years, I had jotted down ideas and anecdotes I intended to use in my books. But the books themselves were all in my head. Arranging them in an orderly fashion on paper—the work part—was a job for which I never found time. Facing Debbie now, the enormity of this loss exploded in my mind, bursting with the sudden realization that life was passing me by.

"Have you published any books?" She asked the question innocently—Debbie always believed I would be a successful writer.

"It's really hard to get published." I said, shrugging my shoulders. The truth of the matter was that I had given up. A multitude of rejection slips had taken their toll. I no longer tried to get published. Writers are supposed to learn to accept rejection, but I never did. I'd lost confidence in my ability to write. I found it easier to bow to rejection and quit than to continue writing.

I was permeated with a bewildering rush of emotions, and I wanted to ignore my feelings of loss. I was a writer who was not writing. And I needed to write. Without my craft, I was dying inside. God had given me a gift that I had rejected by not using it to His glory. By not writing, I denied my very existence—the reason God gave me for being.

In that instant, all the old desires to see my name stamped on the cover of my book were rekindled. Guilt engulfed me. Debbie believed in me as a writer, and I had betrayed that trust by not pursuing the dream. I had let her down. I had let myself down.

We kept the conversation light and upbeat. I hated the clichés that readily sprang to my lips, "How are you doing?" I asked, when I really wanted ask, *Who have you become? Are you still the same sweet, sensitive person I knew on the school bus, or has time calloused you?* Someone once said, "We are the sum total of all of our life experiences."

We chitchatted about her teaching and that she was pursuing a PhD in education and about my writing—or lack of it. We discussed how I happened to find her again after all this time. (I didn't mention why I felt the need to find her now.)

When conversation quickly lagged, I suggested, "Let's go out to the car so you can meet my husband."

As we strolled down the long hallway, engaged in more small talk, I found myself frequently rubbing my forehead and eyes in an effort to restore circulation and clear my mind. My ability to focus and concentrate on her words had become increasingly difficult; my mind seemed to fade in and out of clarity. Fatigue from vacation activities, I decided, had taken its toll on my alertness. Finally, halfway out of the building, I stopped, removed my glasses, and rubbed my eyes and forehead hard, until I could see and think clearly again. It was a gesture I was to remember.

After introducing Debbie to Bud, she gathered her skirt around her legs and sat down on the curb to talk while I stood beside our car. Even this action caught my attention and made we wonder. I, the anemic one, should be fatigued and sitting down, not her. She'd just come from sitting in a meeting. I noticed her ankles were thick and swollen. *Too swollen*, I thought. Did she have kidney disease? Heart disease? High blood pressure? A schoolteacher's ankles from spending too much time on her feet? No, I knew other teachers who didn't have swollen ankles. It couldn't be a school-related affliction.

Our conversation flitted from subject to subject, covering twenty years in twenty minutes. Mostly we talked about what we had done, carefully skirting the real subject: who had we become? How afraid we humans are to share ourselves with each other.

Later, as I reflected on our meeting, I realized, sadly, that I didn't know Debbie anymore. Could we ever recapture the close friendship of our youth? Did we even want to? Our conversation, an attempt to rehash events of our past and fill in the gaps to the present, simply served as an historical overview of our forgotten past. Thomas Wolfe said it best: "You can't go home again."

I left that day feeling sad and deeply troubled. Was it a mistake to destroy this illusion of friendship?

In October 1981, after I discovered I had a hemolytic anemia (not iron deficiency anemia), I learned that Debbie's father had died from liver cancer. Iron overdose (as much as I had received) could manifest itself in liver dysfunction. *Is this the reason*, I wondered, *that God deemed we should meet again? Is my anemia in some way linked to Debbie's father's liver cancer?*

I wrote Debbie, asking for specifics about her father's cancer—a feeble, desperate attempt to find a clue to my own illness.

But she never answered my letters. *How could she be so uncaring about her old friend?* I wondered. (Later, as I faced the possibility of cancer, even the possibility of liver cancer, I understood why God, in His wisdom, spared me the details of that awful disease.)

Even though I received no replies to my letters, I continued to write, reporting the progress of my condition to Debbie as Dr. Fields and I sought to discover a cause for my anemia. Often, I wondered if my problem might be related to an undiagnosed condition in Debbie's body. Why had God arranged our meeting? I was certain it was His doing. The question haunted me. In a strange, unfathomable way, I felt God had given me a responsibility for Debbie but a responsibility I didn't understand.

At other times, I rationalized that the message, "Speak, Lord, for your servant hears," was meant for *me*. Perhaps I only needed this old friend to receive the letters I wrote. This was God's therapy for me as I tried to write out and verbalize this crisis in my life. Once the words were put on paper, the enormity of the problem became more real. I needed to accept my illness and make valuable decisions if, in the final diagnosis, I had cancer—a very real possibility with this type of anemia.

As my worst suspicions about my health became a terrible reality, I blamed Betty, my holistic health practitioner, not so much for the medical half truths she told me but for the complete truths she withheld—the medical facts she held back that made a difference between life or death, her sins of omission.

I agonized about falling victim to the same sin of omission. If God had sent me to warn Debbie, did I dare ignore my assignment? Shouldn't I at least tell her about my concern?

After visiting Dr. Lance in March, Debbie was one of the first persons to whom I wrote. I told her about the mass, the suspicion of cancer, the upcoming liver and kidney scans, and I asked for her prayers. *Prayer*, I thought, *might be the only thing to save me now*. Fear motivated me—fear for myself and fear for my friend. I urged her to consult a gynecologist, if she hadn't already.

"Women over thirty who have never had children are in a high-risk category for developing endometriosis," I wrote, parroting the words of my gynecologist. I enclosed a pamphlet about endometriosis that he had given me.

The week before my surgery, a letter finally arrived from Debbie. Short and succinct, it read, "I do not appreciate your unsolicited medical advice. Do not write me again. Any future letters will be returned." I was stunned and deeply hurt.

Why now? I questioned, rereading the letter. *Why couldn't you wait until after my surgery to dissolve our friendship? Why did you bother to ask for my address if you never intended to write? Why did you hold out hope that our friendship could be rekindled when you never intended to follow through?* Was it just another meaningless gesture of modern times because it seemed like the thing to do at the time—an illusion of friendship that lacked the depth and commitment of real caring?

These and other questions raced through my mind in a tempest of disappointment. Perhaps by *not writing*, she thought she had ended the friendship. Perhaps only I had not gotten the message.

"My God," I cried out in dismay, "what kind of Christian friend has she become?" I would have helped a stranger, and she won't even help a friend. But maybe I wasn't her friend anymore. I thought I was helping her. I wanted to forewarn her. I wanted her to profit from my ignorance. I wanted to *save* her. And I had lost her.

The gift of premonition—was it a blessing or a curse? Rejection washed over me like a polluted wave. Why would anyone believe I had such a gift? Was it even a gift? I knew what I thought about people who claimed to be modern-day prophets or who professed to have the ability to look into the future.

I didn't believe them.

Ironically, Debbie's letter arrived on Monday, the beginning of Holy Week—one week to the day before my surgery. My thoughts turned to Jesus. Jesus too had been betrayed by His trusted friends. How it must have hurt Him. I knelt with Jesus in the Garden of Gethsemane and felt His ache as His friends deserted Him. In His hour of trial, Jesus, too, longed for the love and support of friends, yet His friends deserted Him when they were most needed.

"Could you not watch with me one hour?" Jesus asked. I raged, "Why couldn't you wait until *after my surgery* to write?" Many other close friends also suddenly seemed estranged now—as if cancer was somehow *contagious*.

Months later, I recognized that Debbie's letter was part of God's "great plan." The entire week before surgery I busied myself, mentally berating Debbie for being insensitive, for lacking Christian love and charity. I now accepted all of it as part of God's great diversionary technique. While I spent my internal wrath on Debbie, my external wrath was dissipated with housecleaning, preparing meals to freeze in anticipation of six weeks of inactivity, and fielding phone calls from friends who had not deserted me. Little time remained to fret and worry about the impending surgery.

Like Jesus, I too wished that God would "remove this cup from me." I did not want to experience surgery, but by now I had accepted it as necessary. Still, it was so hard to say, "Not my will, O Lord, but Thine be done." I needed to keep this one thought foremost in my mind. "Not my will, Lord, but Thine be done."

After surgery, when I reflected on the sequence of events, I thought, *If only I could blame Debbie. If only I could hate her.* Perhaps then accepting the pain of losing her would be easier, less bitter. But I could not. Because when I was painfully honest with myself, I knew who had destroyed our friendship—*and it wasn't Debbie.*

Oh, the temporal temptation to *be* God, instead of to *serve* Him.

And I wept. I wept for a friendship forever lost in the intangible tangle of time. I wept for my friend, and I wept for myself and for man's inhumanity to man, which allows us—through our own ignorance and insensitivity and because of our own needs and fears—to ignore the needs and fears of others.

What right did I have to call myself *friend*? What right did I have to throw stones? In my heart, Debbie would always be *my* friend; I just wasn't *her* friend anymore.

Some months later, Mom mailed me a newspaper clipping that announced Debbie's marriage. She had found that special man to share her life.

And I found my muse. I joined a Christian writers' club and became a freelance writer, publishing articles, short stories, poetry, and humorous fillers in more than one hundred different magazines and newspapers in the United States and Canada.

God puts special people in our lives at certain critical times for special purposes.

CHAPTER 13

TWO FRIENDS: THE NEW

"God never closes a door but that He opens a window." An older neighbor friend often quoted these words to me when we met for coffee. The words more often seemed to rationalize some misfortune or disappointment in her own life than to give me advice. Now, the words returned to comfort me with new clarity and understanding.

With Debbie, my door was closing; with Laura, my new spiritual friend, my window was opening.

Just as I believed God foreordained my chance encounter with Debbie, I also believed God's master plan intended that I meet Laura, who was selected to fill a spiritual-friendship void in my life. We can never begin to imagine or anticipate the multitude of ways God comes into our lives to care for us.

Curiously, the same qualities that endeared Debbie to me also attracted me to Laura. Unmistakably intelligent, Laura was a warm, sensitive, caring person. We became acquainted at a Christian women's executive board meeting. Even though I was the newly appointed editor of the organization's newsletter, I lacked her self-assurance. Laura was an *elected* member to the board.

Preparation of the quarterly publication, *The Communicator*, was a task I looked forward to with both joy and trepidation. I knew I possessed the necessary typing and layout skills, but I lacked spiritual commitment and savvy.

When first approached about the job of editor, I resisted, believing it would require too much time away from my husband and my home. The basis of my resistance, however, involved my lack of commitment. I simply did not want to get involved.

Involvement demands time. Involvement demands energy. Involvement demands sharing oneself. *I didn't want to get involved.*

But God wanted me involved. He had given me a gift, and I was not using that gift for His purpose—or for any purpose—at that time. Since leaving the advertising field to become a full-time housewife and helpmate, I had quit writing creatively. I had buried my light under a bushel and turned my back on the bushel.

But God has a master plan for each of our lives. In my master plan was the requirement that I begin writing again. He started me with something easy; something at which He knew I could succeed—a quarterly religious newsletter. I didn't even have to write the articles; I only edited, typed, prepared a layout with clip artwork, and pasted up the finished newsletter so it could be copied. Someone else printed and distributed it.

That I should meet and be befriended by Laura, when I most needed a deeply spiritual friend, was a bonus.

It was not the first time our paths had crossed. At the organization's district fall convention, Laura conducted a workshop that I attended. At the time, she suffered from an undiagnosed physical disability that caused her to conduct the seminar from a chair. When she asked for someone to serve as her blackboard secretary, I volunteered.

Even ill, Laura was a dynamic, forceful person. Her exuberance and knowledge were contagious, as was her interest and devotion to her subject. This mentally energetic woman fascinated me. Later, other board members told me Laura had considerable status as a knowledgeable expert in her field—energy: nuclear and alternative sources.

While some Christians picketed and chanted, "Stop the growth of nuclear power plants," Laura campaigned to build more worldwide. Her reasoning: countries that lack energy do not flourish. They often revert to the lowest forms of survival. Energy sources are the one necessity most undeveloped nations lack. Energy is vital for producing food and other basic necessities of life. "Without energy," Laura contended, "nations do not develop and progress to their full potential. People perish from the destructive effects of energy shortages."

I admired Laura for championing an unpopular cause. She had not reached her conclusions blindly, as did many people who opposed nuclear power. Laura studied, traveled, researched, and talked to experts in the field of energy. She knew her facts, and when you heard her speak or talked to her, you were persuaded by her knowledge and authority.

Laura often referred to herself as a "professional volunteer"—a person who does for free what other people are paid to do. Married and the mother of four grown children, she said they were the reason she expressed interest in the energy future of our country and the world.

She believed nuclear power should and could be harnessed for the public good, often quoting 1 Timothy 4:4 RSV—"For everything created by God is good, and nothing is to be rejected if it is received with thanksgiving"

"Mankind," she explained, "is simply charged with the responsibility to use it for good purposes and to share this knowledge with all the peoples of the world. Part of our human task is to find a way to neutralize the harmful waste products that concern so many people."

She believed it wasn't nuclear power or even nuclear pollution that frightened the general public; they feared the unknown. Uncertainty about the future effect these nuclear waste products could have on their lives—and on the lives of their children and grandchildren—was among their biggest concerns. Man's fear was of the unknown future.

As I faced an unknown, undiagnosed illness, I could relate to those fears. It takes a stalwart Christian, firm in faith and courage, to face fear and uncertainty, secure in the knowledge that with God's help, all things are possible. Christians must be a people set apart, willing to take firm, unpopular stands, if the world is to benefit.

Laura was a natural teacher, and because I was a writer and journalist and an inquisitive person, I wanted to learn from her. It wasn't an effort; it became an enjoyable, enlightening experience.

Until we became better acquainted, I admired Laura from afar, as well as admiring her persistence and courage to pursue what she believed to be truth. But her warm, sensitive, and caring nature drew me to her as a friend—a trait I found all too rare in the world today.

Although I greatly admired Laura as a leader, by this time in my life I knew how spiritually dangerous it is to make gods out of people. While God will not disappoint us if we remember that all things are planned according to His will and purpose, people do disappoint us. Sometimes the disappointment can be devastating, especially when we endow them with qualities they do not intrinsically possess. Hero worship is dangerous, yet some people cultivate it. They thrive on the adulation of others—lesser beings than themselves, of course. It is just as destructive to be the hero worshipper, putting yourself on a lower plane, as it is to covet the worship, putting yourself on the higher plane. We are all one in God.

People fall from the pedestals upon which we place them. They sin. Sometimes they sin against us, their worshippers, but gods aren't supposed to sin, so we reject them—the gods we have made of them. And in the process, we lose the friendship of many good people.

Although I admired Laura, I recognized her humanity. I knew that sometime in our relationship, she would disappoint me. And I would disappoint her. I would be required to forgive her, and she would need to forgive me. For thoughtlessness? For inconsistency? I didn't know what, but I knew forgiveness would be required because we both were human.

In the early 1980's, about the time I met Laura, a new humanist movement was sweeping our country and the world. It taught humankind to make gods of *people*, so we wouldn't have to forgive each other. It eliminated the need for forgiveness by eliminating sin. Thus, it also eliminated our need for Jesus, our savior from sin. The Antichrist movement was alive and growing – it promoted the illusion of perfection and control; that man could be a perfect human being in control of his own life and future. It was a false illusion that implied we didn't need God or Jesus Christ--that humans could save themselves. Unfortunately, what the movement professed was only an illusion of truth. It was a new age, but the same old lies that had trapped humans in the past. Like looking for the pot of gold at the end of the rainbow, people who subscribed to this ideology chased a dream that could never be realized.

I shared no such illusions about Laura. I accepted her with her faults. And she accepted me with my burdens.

The executive board met in November 1981, just two weeks after my first visit to the hematologist. By now, I knew I did not have iron deficiency anemia, yet something was terribly wrong with my body. Worry about my unknown illness gripped me. And rage held me in its clutches; rage that was directed against the holistic medical staff that had so easily and completely deceived me into believing I could control my health. While they profited, my medical condition deteriorated.

Laura and I attended the fall executive board meeting, where we became reacquainted. At times, my mind felt muddled and foggy from what I now believe to be from iron and vitamin overdose. Often, there seemed to be a two- or three-minute delay between the time I heard verbal information and when I could process it into my brain. Some information wasn't being entered at all. I felt that I assimilated only half of what I heard. Inwardly, I seethed with anger against the holistic practitioners who had so easily deluded me.

That morning, another board member, Nancy, led devotions. She asked each of the twenty women at the meeting to draw a floor plan of their spiritual house, using the crayons and paper provided. Each house should include a specific number of rooms—the library (a study of the mind), the dining room (our appetites and desires), the living room (where friends gather, our fellowship area), the workroom (where we use our talents and skills), the playroom (what do we do for fun), and the closets (whatever we were hiding).

After our spiritual houses were drawn, we gathered in small groups of four or five to share our plans. One of the rules was that we didn't have to share anything we didn't want to share. I waited until everyone else had shared, and when attention turned toward me, I announced, "I must have been daydreaming when the instructions were given. My house isn't at all like the rest of yours." I folded my floor plan in half, tucked it into my Bible, and refused to share any part of it.

Laura was in my group; only she noticed and responded to the conflict raging within my soul. Before returning to our seats, she said to me, "I think you need a hug," and she enveloped me in a warm embrace.

I did need a hug. The assurance that someone else shared my conflict comforted me. The spontaneous gesture brought tears to my eyes, and although grateful for her recognition and response, I couldn't bring myself to tell her why I had refused to share my floor plan. Still, I knew I needed a confidant, a spiritually based person with whom I could express my problems, my frustrations, and my fears. I needed the counsel of someone who was concerned but not closely allied with me; someone who could look at my situation with an objective, dispassionate viewpoint and could listen while I sorted out a course of action.

I especially needed someone in whom to confide my fears, which I didn't even want to admit existed. Fears I refused to tell my husband or my parents, lest I cause them unnecessary anguish. But fears that had to be addressed so decisions could be made. Fears about cancer and its consequences. Fears about death.

Laura, knowingly or unknowingly, entered into this fellowship of suffering with me. According to biblical admonition, she elected to share my burdens.

Though concerned and curious, she did not question or pry into the reasons for my strange behavior that weekend. Her eyes followed me, patiently waiting for me to share a clue, a hint about the problem that held me prisoner. But I could not share. I could neither reveal nor express the rage bottled inside. Yet her unvoiced concern told me that God had designed my support network.

Our devotional project for the next morning was to redesign our spiritual houses. This time we were to make it a dream house—a house we could be proud to have God visit. We had all day and night to think about the ideal spiritual plan for our lives.

That night, as I lay awake, pondering my floor plan, I suddenly realized what my spiritual house lacked. My closets were a mess—the areas where we hide the things we don't want others to see. What was I hiding in mine? My trust! Trust—the one thing I should be scattering throughout my living area—was locked safely away in my spiritual closet. Why was I keeping it there?

The next morning at devotions, instead of returning to our small groups, we shared our new floor plans with everyone. I felt decidedly more confident now after revamping my spiritual floor plan. My new house was built without closets. There would be no place to hide my trust. And my new house included a lot of windows and a skylight to let in God's warmth and understanding. Last, I put a broom in every room—to sweep away the cobwebs of doubt, despair, and uncertainty that I knew would return to clutter my spirituality. For the first time since hearing the hematologist's pronouncement, I looked to the future with hope and trust.

After returning to Phoenix, I wrote Laura a long letter, summarizing my anemia problems—my "own energy crisis," as I had come to term it. I told her about the unexplained, abnormal cells found in my bone marrow. The reason I had said nothing at the board meeting, I explained, was because I didn't know anything, for sure. I didn't even know if I had a real problem, adding that by the next board meeting, six months hence, perhaps the problem would be resolved or at least diagnosed.

I mailed Laura periodic medical reports as new blood tests ruled out different disorders, while the cause of the low red-cell count remained a mystery. Unlike Debbie, Laura expressed concern and curiosity. But like Debbie, she did not write letters. Occasionally, though, she called long distance from California.

In February, Laura was scheduled to give her energy talk to our church women's group. I invited her to stay overnight with us. Her return flight was scheduled for late the next day. God provided an opportunity for us to visit.

I shared my blood problems in detail with her, as well as my frustrations at not finding a quicker solution. As an encouraging and sympathetic listener, she shared her own problems and frustrations of the previous year when she sought to uncover elusive medical answers. Her problem was hypoglycemia—low blood sugar. It took a nine-hour glucose tolerance test to detect it. I was well acquainted with hypoglycemia, having been diagnosed sixteen years earlier, so I could relate to her frustration.

In her younger years, Laura also had been diagnosed with anemia and admitted she took iron occasionally, even now, for fatigue. She was understandably interested in my findings about iron overdose and the problems it caused. Had God brought us together so I could warn her about the dangers of iron overdose?

Laura and I shared mutual concerns. More than similar health problems, we shared a spiritual reinforcement. We both knew that no matter how much we willed ourselves to be well and whole again, our will would not be done unless God willed it too. Laura provided Christian support and reassurance, which was invaluable to me as I began my quest for truth. What was God's will for my life?

Laura didn't offer advice. She listened. She became a sounding board, someone to whom I could express the fears and doubts that constantly percolated in my mind. She didn't judge or criticize me for lack of faith, nor did she dismiss my fears as unfounded. She listened, allowing me to make my own decisions, confident that with God's help, the right decision would be made.

Laura said she would be praying for me, and I knew that she did—I *felt* the prayers. Peace began to creep into my life.

Unlike Debbie, Laura didn't leave me alone in total silence, lonely and ignored. She voiced concern through mutual friends and, as mentioned, occasional long-distance phone calls.

When my gynecologist recommended an immediate hysterectomy

because cancer might be lurking in my body, Laura was among the first persons I told. *Cancer*—I needed to face the possibility. *Cancer*. If it was in my body, what did I intend to do about it? *Cancer*. Should I opt for surgery and risk spreading it, or should I refuse surgery and opt for death with dignity?

As my doctors sought to confirm or eliminate cancer as the source of my symptoms, I became a frequent visitor to the nuclear medicine section of Mercy General Hospital. How much radioactivity did I receive? Could it damage my body? Would I click if I walked past a Geiger counter?

Conversations with Laura reassured me. She explained that radiation exposure from low-level x-rays used for diagnostic purposes were less harmful than the scaremongers would have the public believe. The benefits derived from early detection and treatment of disease far outweighed the slight risks from overexposure. A competent doctor would not request unnecessary tests.

I prayed that she was right.

In the beginning, when I visited the hematologist and gynecologist, I told both doctors I wanted to know everything. I didn't want any surprises. Although I do not regret that decision, at times it caused unnecessary mental anguish. I can understand why doctors sometimes are reluctant to share all test results with their patients, especially when later tests rule out suspected problems.

When Laura received my letter, written out of fear and desperation about the cancer possibility, she tried to call me at home, but I was at the hospital, undergoing kidney and liver scans. So she called a fellow board member, a member of my church, who knew nothing definite at that time, as I knew nothing.

After months of inaction, events were beginning to move fast—too fast. I imagined being on a medical merry-go-round—only I couldn't get off.

Two days later, after receiving the results of the liver and kidney scans, I wrote to Laura reporting the findings and giving her the surgery date—one week before our spring board meeting. Indeed, it seemed the problem was being resolved before the board was to meet again.

Before receiving my latest letter, Laura phoned me at home. I apologized for causing her undue concern but was reassured by her concern, expressed in a tangible way. Her phone call showed her interest above and beyond the call of Christian duty and provided added—and needed—spiritual support. Laura shared experiences about her relatives who had fought cancer and, with God's grace, had achieved temporary victory. All victories over death are only temporary.

Her testimony provided the extra strength I needed to give up and give God the opportunity to work His miracles in my life, to let God decide if my life on earth, my purpose for being, was finished. If only we all could be "little Christs" in our daily ministering.

After surgery, during my recovery period, while others sent flowers and cards, Laura sent Lloyd Ogilvie's book *Life without Limits: The Message of Mark's Gospel.*[7] It was the beginning of a daily journey into God's Word. As I delved deeper and deeper into scripture, I realized how starved my soul had become for God's Word. How deep the void is when one is lost without God's hope.

At the time, I didn't understand why my search of the scriptures often took me to the book of 1 John 4. I read and reread that chapter. "Test the spirits to see whether they are of God; for many false prophets have gone out into the world." Was God helping me to remove the influence of holistic medicine from my life? I desperately clung to the promise found in verse 1 John 4:18. "Perfect love casts out fear."

Debbie helped me to realize that I wasn't making time to use my God-given gift, but Laura led me to realize I wasn't making time in my life for God.

As I filled my soul with scripture, the rage within me quieted to resolution. Did I hold the key to exposing holistic medicine? Had God put me in the wrong place for the right reason?

---

[7] Lloyd J. Ogilvie. *Life without Limits: The Message of Mark's Gospel* (Waco, Tex.: Word Books, 1975).

If I did hold the key, I knew God could show me the way. He had been busy teaching me patience and trust. This time, I would let Him set the timetable, and it would be perfect.

Years later, as I reflected on these experiences, putting them and the outcome into proper perspective, I was finally able to ask myself which friend had taught me the most about God and love and forgiveness, and which friend had taught me the most about myself as a person, a friend, and a Christian.

They both did. We learn about God from everyone we meet, if we look for God in our fellow humans. Jesus said, "Truly, I say to you, as you did it to one of the least of these my brethren, you did it to me" (Matthew 25:40 RSV).

Because one friend sought out me, a lost and frightened creature, and loved me through the hurting, I was able to put God's loving forgiveness into practice with the other friend. God meets us through people. Christians must be involved in *doing* the Word—healing hurts by forgiving each other. We must find the Lord's lost sheep and love them back into the flock. It can't be a group round-up. The strays—God's hurting people—must be found one by one. We must become attuned to the bleat of the lost sheep needing help that God sends our way. Christianity must be practiced on a person-to-person basis.

"Whoever brings back a sinner from the error of his way will save his soul from death and will cover a multitude of sins" (James 5:20 RSV). Nothing happens in life but that God expects good to come from it. "Old things are passed away; behold, all things are become new" (2 Corinthians 5:17 KJV).

CHAPTER 14

"YOU DIDN'T HAVE THE PAIN"

On the Tuesday before my surgery, I stopped at the local library and checked out three books: two on hysterectomy and one on cancer chemotherapy. Although the hysterectomy books brought new insights, I found little written—especially in layman's language—about ovarian cancer and its treatments. Rather than chemotherapy for ovarian cancer, most doctors recommended radiation treatment. But these books were several years old; new technologies were being introduced every day.

I tried to keep busy. I suppose Bud thought he was being helpful when he suggested I clean up both my work room and our game room so I wouldn't accidentally trip over clutter when I returned home from the hospital. "I only have *one week* before surgery," I replied. "You are asking the impossible."

I picked up our airplane tickets to Minneapolis for the July wedding of my niece, Elaine. I wanted to have them in hand if I should not be allowed to drive after surgery. I also purchased a two-inch-thick foam pad for the twin bed in the spare bedroom where I'd be sleeping during recovery. Van, my sister-in-law, had had a hysterectomy the year before; she said the extra padding would feel good.

It was interesting to get phone calls and letters from Christian friends. Some seemed more anxious about my surgery than I was. Others were concerned because they thought I might be frightened. When they learned I was not afraid, their attitudes changed and they were more upbeat in their support; others didn't seem to comprehend that a person could face serious surgery and *not* be afraid. Perhaps their faith had never been tested like this.

In times of crisis, I found that talking with people who were uplifting in their outlook made a big difference in how I felt about talking to them. I appreciated the friends who felt that God's will would be done and who reminded me of that promise. This common spiritual bond brought closeness between us.

I was surprised and gratified by the new relationships I forged with like-minded friends, as well as the relationships that were strained because we had no spiritual closeness. Many of the women on the district executive board became very dear to me, while some members of my church congregation became spiritual strangers.

On Wednesday, I woke feeling melancholy. Before beginning my daily housework, I decided to read a few chapters from *And a Time to Live: Toward Emotional Well-Being During the Crisis of Cancer*[8] by Robert Chernin Cantor. The author spoke of "preparatory mourning" and "anticipatory mourning." At times, I felt the need for a good cry but couldn't seem to get started. My eyes filled with tears, but I couldn't bring the emotions any closer to the surface. According to one authority, this is the process of "weeping"—a form of mourning. It was totally out of character for me; I'd never been a weeper or a crier, and I couldn't imagine what I might be mourning—certainly not the end of my menstrual periods. My menstrual period was due any day—could it be premenstrual blues?

On Thursday, I woke to pain and a throbbing ache in my left side. Now that I knew the mass was there, I imagined I could feel it pressing if I lay a certain way or turned to an unusual position.

Two separate friends invited me for coffee. I accepted both invitations, one in the morning and the other in the afternoon. Although

---

[8] Robert Chernin Cantor. *And a Time to Live: Toward Emotional Well-Being During the Crisis of Cancer* (New York: HarperCollins, 1980).

it interrupted my housecleaning activities, the quiet support of Mary and Irene was uplifting.

Friday, April 9, 1982—Good Friday

Even though I try to convince myself that I'm not worried about the surgery, I know that subconsciously I am. Last night I dreamed I was buying large quantities of chicken—saving and freezing all the livers because I knew I would have to provide my own liver replacement during surgery. Size didn't seem to matter as much as quantity.

At three o'clock this afternoon, I had such an intense feeling of sadness that I went into the bedroom and cried, sobbing into a pillow to muffle the sounds. I didn't want to upset Mitzi, our little cocker spaniel mix. I'm *not afraid* of the surgery, but I guess I'm *scared*. Today I had another premonition: "Don't worry about this operation; the cancer is *not* in your ovaries."

Where is it then? I questioned, but the telepathy that brought the message offered no further information.

So I guess I'm still scared, afraid that although the surgery will correct the ureter deviation, the *real cancer* lurks somewhere else in my body, still undetected.

On Saturday, I awoke in extreme pain. It felt like the mass growing inside me was getting ready to explode. But within an hour, the pain had subsided.

Bud and I went to a fancy restaurant that night. I had lobster—one of my favorite meals—and was glad that I wasn't allergic to iodine. Bud teased me about eating my "last supper," although I knew I would get supper at the hospital the following night.

On the way home, Bud admitted to being glad the "waiting and worrying" would soon be over—his first and only indication that he was worried about my surgery. During the past several weeks, his attitude seemed so positive, almost to the point of denial, I thought. He *expected* the surgical outcome to be successful—meaning benign.

That night I started my period. I comforted myself with the thought, *If my cycle runs true to form, with the second day, Monday, being the most painful, by then I'll be having surgery and, hopefully, won't feel a thing.*

On Easter Sunday, the day before surgery, I woke at 4:00 a.m. with severe abdominal pain. Emptying my bladder helped, but my period had arrived with all its fury. I wanted to spend this last morning in bed, lying with Bud's arms around me, holding me. I knew he needed the closeness as much as I did, especially today. But I *hurt so much.* I hurt all over. The pain started in front, in my abdomen, and circled my entire body. My pelvic bones ached. My kidneys hurt. The abdominal cramping came in painful undulating waves that rose and fell. I hurt so much I didn't want Bud to even *touch* me. I told him so he wouldn't wonder why I pulled away. I just wanted to lie quietly until the cramping passed. Eventually, the pain grew less. I got up, washed, brushed my teeth, dressed, and took Mitzi for her morning walk. The pain was now only moderate. How does one measure and describe pain?

We went to the eight o'clock Easter morning service. I neglected to empty my bladder before leaving the house and regretted it halfway through the service, as I suffered much pain from pressure on the bladder. *Is it menstrual pain or cancer pain?* I wondered. Pain is so vague. Several times I considered leaving the service to go to the bathroom, but then the pain would temporarily subside, and I would decide to tough it out a little while longer. I was glad to be having the surgery, if only to get rid of this monthly ordeal. I would not miss the pain.

My mind wandered to a conversation I'd had with Bud's dad after his open-heart surgery ten years earlier. The doctors had given him only a fifty-fifty chance of surviving the surgery. I had remarked, "With those odds, I'm not sure I would have opted for surgery."

His simple response: "*You* didn't have the pain." Today, I had the pain and, like him, I longed for the relief that surgery would bring.

I didn't hear much of the Easter sermon. I wondered if one of the three pastors would visit me in the hospital before my surgery to check on my spiritual well-being. To date, none had called to offer spiritual support to Bud or me, not even to inquire if we were spiritually prepared for this surgery. They knew my surgery was scheduled and that cancer was suspected because I had put myself on the prayer list. *Sadly, the more pastors we add to the church staff,* I thought, *the more ministry seems to be neglected.*

At 2:00 p.m., I checked into the hospital. Pre-op testing included a chest x-ray, more blood tests, and a 12-lead EKG. At 3:00 p.m., I got into my room, with instructions to give a "clean catch" urine sample. Two different nurses took my medical history.

Linda O'Toole, the swing-shift nurse, a very pleasant person, seemed to have a lot of time to visit. Had she had been instructed to calm down preoperative patients? I felt very calm.

My roommate, Sara, arrived at 4:30 p.m. Linda asked if Sara was allergic to iodine. She was. I thought, *It's a good thing I'm not allergic since no one asked me about an iodine allergy.* But perhaps they already knew I wasn't allergic from the liver and kidney scans already performed—I'd been given iodine infusions for both of them.

Sara also was scheduled for a hysterectomy and was anything but calm. I understood why when I learned she'd almost bled to death during a previous surgery.

By contrast, I could hardly believe how calm I felt, like I was standing outside my body, watching this drama unfold, as if I were a spectator instead of the participant.

The reason for my calmness had to be the prayers of support from all over the country—from my family and my local and church friends, as well as the members of my district executive board. Many times we don't get needed prayer support because we are unable to share our fears and ask for it. "You do not have, because you do not ask" (James 4:2 RSV). I shared my fears with almost everyone I knew and asked for their prayers. Now the prayers were coming back to bless me. It felt comforting to know I was not alone. God had wrapped me safely in His arms of love. I wasn't afraid.

Dr. Lewis, the hospital intern, took my case history (again) and examined me. I quizzed him about the pain in my shin bone. He reassured me. "It's probably *not* malignant. It's not in the right place for bone cancer." Dr. Lance later confirmed that observation.

"You have what we call a 'virgin' tummy," Dr. Lewis commented, trying to put me at ease while checking my abdomen. I told him what Bud had said about it not being "virgin" anymore. We both laughed. He checked my breasts. "The lumpiness isn't in a part of the breast that is normally malignant," he told me, "unless it occurs in both breasts—and yours doesn't. Watch for hardening of the lumps, dimpling of the breasts, discharge from the nipples, or other unusual changes."

I hoped that with all the prayer support I had received that the mass would have miraculously disappeared, and surgery would not be needed, but the pelvic exam proved otherwise. It was still there and still painful when touched.

Dr. Lance arrived about 6:00 p.m. I had another typed page of questions to ask and was glad that he had interrupted his Easter to schedule this final presurgical visit.

"Will you explain the calcium deposits in my abdomen one more time?" I asked. "How serious are they? Will they complicate the surgery?"

"You don't have to worry about them," he replied. "When we did the kidney pyelogram, which also scans the abdomen, they had disappeared."

"Might I have a 'chocolate' [blood-filled] cyst?" I asked.

"There is a fifty-fifty chance that it is," he answered.

I had read about blood-filled cysts. They were not cancerous. This was the most hope that I had received. I wondered if that type of cyst also might explain the anemia.

"The pain," he said, "might be caused by adhesions—the growing together of the various internal organs with endometriosis—pulling on each other."

"Does recovery from endometriosis take longer to heal than a regular hysterectomy?" I asked.

"Usually not. It depends on the patient and the amount of surgery."

"What will you do if cancer is found?"

"If the tumor is malignant, we will biopsy other nearby organs and remove any cancerous lumps found, whether on the bowel, bladder, or other organs." He reassured me they would not remove complete organs. The recommended treatment was chemotherapy. *Personally*, I thought, *I'd prefer chemo to radiation.*

"I don't have any swollen glands in the groin area," I said. "Is that a good sign?"

"The lymph nodes that would swell are internal, not external."

"If it is cancer, will you do a radical hysterectomy?" From my reading, I learned that a radical hysterectomy involved removing all the associated lymph glands.

"If malignant, they would be removed," he said.

"Can I get a copy of your surgical report and the pathologist's report?"

"That can be arranged."

Our meeting took less than fifteen minutes. He said he would see me in the morning before surgery and urged me to take the sleeping pill to get a good night's rest.

After he left, the nurse prepped me for surgery. She shaved me from pelvis to breast, although I couldn't imagine finding body hair that high. I dreaded the itching from the regrowth of hair after surgery but found that was one of the lesser postsurgery discomforts.

At eight o'clock, I received instructions for turning over properly after surgery. At nine o'clock, I got an enema and vaginal douche. Then came the surgical shower. The area where the incision would be made had to be scrubbed vigorously with soap for several minutes. Finally, I felt clean, inside and out.

Since my period had started, I'd brought along my own sanitary napkins and belt. After surgery, however, I was advised I would need to use hospital supplies; everything had to be sterile after surgery. "You can use your supplies when you return home." Nurse Linda informed me there would be some bleeding and discharge for a while afterward.

Linda also urged me to move, wiggle my toes, and do the deep breathing and coughing exercises outlined in the postoperative surgical care guide. The deep breathing and coughing exercises were to help get the anesthetic out of my lungs. Wiggling my toes and moving helped to prevent blood clots from forming. "Do not cross your legs after surgery," she cautioned, "as that causes the blood to pool and allows clots to form." There were so many things to remember. I wondered if I would recall everything when I was doped up.

Since I wasn't allergic to iodine, I received a vaginal gel to treat infections—perhaps as a preventive measure because of my menstrual period. At 10:30 p.m., the nurse brought a sleeping pill. No pastor from my church had visited or called. *What did I expect?* I thought. *It's Easter. They have their own families.* Still, I was disappointed. My doctor had interrupted his Easter to care for my physical and emotional needs, but my pastor showed no concern for my spiritual needs. *Why are we supporting this church?* I wondered.

I slept soundly. At 5:30 a.m., I awoke and brushed my teeth. I wanted to be ready for Bud's early morning visit.

CHAPTER 15

SURGERY

Bud arrived at the hospital at 5:50 a.m. His dad, who planned to sit with him during surgery, came with him.

"Did any of the pastors visit you last night?" Bud asked.

"No," I responded. "I didn't really expect them to. A phone call would have been nice, though."

I put on a special surgical gown, got the sedative shot about 6:30 a.m., and was moved to a gurney. Bud and Pa followed the gurney to the operating room waiting area. I felt very relaxed. Neither of them talked, so I chattered all the way down what seemed like miles of corridor. I felt unbelievably calm and peaceful—and unafraid. I wanted to relay that feeling to them.

Bud kissed me at the door. My gurney was wheeled into a large operating waiting room. Three or four other people on gurneys were already neatly lined up along the wall. The attendant wheeled me to a place in line. *Will they take us in the order in which we're lined up?* I wondered.

The cool room might have seemed chilly to me under normal circumstances, but the relaxing shot I had been given began to take effect. I felt warm and pleasant. One more gurney came into the waiting room before I was wheeled into the operating room. One gurney that was there when I first arrived still remained. They *weren't* taking us in order.

Compared to the huge waiting area, the operating room looked tiny, much smaller than I expected. The battery of high-powered lights overhead seemed to cover half of the operating room's ceiling. They appeared to hang so low that I wondered if the doctors would bump their heads on them if they stood up. They probably avoided colliding with the lights because most of the time they were bending over the patient.

Dr. Lance entered the OR, greeted me, and introduced his associate, who would be assisting. The anesthesiologist introduced himself. "We'll be starting soon," Dr. Lance said.

The last thing I remember was Dr. Lance's handsome, reassuring smile. I wanted to let him know that I was at peace and okay with the surgery.

"I'm not afraid," I said. And I wasn't. I knew I had found a doctor I could trust. I started to count backward. One hundred, ninety-nine, ninety-eight, ninety-seven, ninety-six …

The next thing I heard was Dr. Lance whispering the sweetest words in my ear, "It's all right, June. No cancer." Then I was out again. For the first time in years, I felt no pain.

Later, Bud told me I'd left the operating room at 9:30 a.m. Surgery had lasted approximately ninety minutes. At 11:00 a.m., having returned to my hospital room, I vaguely remember Bud reassuring me. "There was no cancer, baby. Everything was benign." And I replied, "Yes, I know." My words were thick and heavy from the drugs. Speaking was an effort.

The remainder of the day was hazy. I drifted in and out of dreamland, waking occasionally, feeling the need to urinate. Then, seeing the catheter and urine bag, I remembered I was not allowed to get out of bed.

The next day, Bud told me he had reassured me there was no cancer every time I woke up, but I only remembered his telling me one time. Apparently my drugged reply, "Yes, I know," went unvoiced.

Van, my sister-in-law, also sat with Bud and Pa during and after the surgery. Harriet Hammon, our older neighbor and friend from church, came to my room later to bring an Easter lily from church. I had no recollection of seeing either Van or Harriet.

The one person I remembered seeing was my hematologist, Dr. Fields. He looked so tall but always stood bent over at the shoulders. *Because of his height?* I wondered. He peered down at me, solemn and grave. Was he part of a drug-induced dream? Or was he real?

He came to visit the next day when I was awake. "Did you stop by to see me yesterday afternoon?" I asked. He confirmed he had visited. Having two such caring physicians cheered me.

The first evening I received a pain shot every three hours and became more conscious of activity around me. Every light in the room blazed so brightly that I thought it was daytime. Every time I woke up, I imagined another day had passed. I continually asked the nurse, "What day is it? What time is it? Is it morning or night?" I couldn't comprehend that the time passing was only a few hours.

The nurses were pleased with my progress. Even in my drugged state, I heard them commenting, "She's turning over by herself already." I couldn't bear to lie in one position very long but found that by turning myself over, the nurses lost track of which hip should get the next shot, and sometimes I got two shots in a row in the same hip. I wasn't coherent enough to make them understand it was the other hip's turn.

Every time a nurse entered the room, she said, "Wiggle your toes." Once during that first night I woke up in pain. Usually when I rang, I got a shot, and the pain dissolved into sleep. But this time the nurse said, "You have to wait another half hour." Time flew by; I don't think I was ever completely conscious. I floated in a twilight zone.

I awoke the next day feeling miraculously refreshed and well rested. Bud stopped on his way to work. Dr. Lance came in and told us about the surgery.

"The cyst on your left ovary," he said, "was as large as a grapefruit—a very large grapefruit." He indicated the size with his cupped hands. "It was filled with water and blood—a chocolate cyst. If it had burst before surgery, it would have been like a burst appendix, only it would have been ten times more dangerous because of its size. If you'd been taken to the hospital in an emergency situation, you probably would have died from peritonitis before we could have identified the source of the problem and gone in surgically to save you. As it turned out, the cyst did break when we were removing it, but we were ready for that. We did copious irrigations to rid your body of infection." Now I understood why a biopsy of the cyst would not have been wise.

Betty's words came back to haunt me: *"Once you reach menopause, everything will dry up and go away."* With new insight, I realized I probably never would have reached menopause—the cyst could have burst at any time. Fortunately, Dr. Lance had scheduled surgery before it ruptured. Now I understood why both Dr. Fields and Dr. Lance were so anxious to book surgery immediately.

It finally dawned on me—my holistic caregivers didn't care if I lived. How could they be so callous? They knew this cyst would kill me if it wasn't removed, but dead patients tell no tales. Anger and rage filled my being and crept down into my soul.

Dr. Lance further explained that the endometriosis had caused all the pain. The blood-filled cyst, an infectious cyst, had resulted from the endometriosis. The left fallopian tube was completely fused shut by endometrial growth, and the right fallopian tube was so inflamed that it soon would have been fused shut too. There was no way I could have gotten pregnant with two obstructed fallopian tubes.

The cyst completely blocked the left fallopian tube, pressing on the left ureter, the tube that delivers urine from the kidney to the bladder. The ureter, while not completely blocked, was badly kinked. Untreated, it could have soon caused kidney failure. Dr. Lance reported he had had to do a lot of "reconstructive" work on it, scraping the ureter to rid it of attached endometriosis. This caused both the ureter and left kidney to be severely traumatized. That explained the blood in my urine—I had noticed red in the catheter urine bag.

"The adhesions, or scar tissue from the endometriosis, were extensive.

I had to practically peel your bladder," he said, adding that adhesions were also on the bowel. "The bowel wall was not yet penetrated, but if left untreated it probably would have necessitated a bowel resection. We did a lot of cutting. You'll probably be sore for quite a while."

Compared to the pain I'd suffered in past years, I experienced surprisingly little pain now and wondered if this was God's hand working in my body. The one thing I'd most prayed for was freedom from pain. Later, I realized the pain shots were keeping me free from immediate pain.

Earlier, Bud told me Dr. Lance had also checked the gall bladder and liver during the exploratory procedure. The liver was normal—smooth and slippery, no lumps or growths. The gall bladder contained no stones. The liver concerned me because of the risk of damage from iron overdose, so this new knowledge gave me peace of mind. Dr. Lance reaffirmed the liver findings, adding he had also removed my appendix because it was easy to reach. "We won't have to worry about it if you have more pain in that area." He said he'd ordered a hormone shot after surgery. "It should last about two weeks." The hormone shot would replace the estrogen that the ovaries normally would produce. Later, he would prescribe estrogen replacement in pill form.

As I improved, I noticed my right hip felt completely numb. Dr. Lewis, the hospital resident, explained, "This happens sometimes when nerves are severed during the incision. They might regenerate in six months, or you might always have the numbness."

I remembered that when Bud had skin cancers removed from his forehead he'd experienced numbness because of severed nerves, but they regenerated in three or four months. It was not something unique to my surgery.

The nurse encouraged me to cough frequently, saying, "Place a pillow over the incision whenever you cough." I noticed now that my incision only extended to the belly button. Although securely fastened with what looked like huge metal staples, I feared my incision might pop open at any time, and all my internal organs would come tumbling out. Rationally, I knew that was impossible, but it was an abnormal fear for the first week or two. Because of the incision, my abdominal walls felt fragile.

Sneezing was a terrible experience. I tried to stifle sneezes as much as possible; I was afraid it would open the incision. My throat was sore and raw. At first, I blamed sinus drainage for my throat discomfort, but my nurse said more likely it was from the breathing tube that had been inserted down my throat during surgery. As she predicted, the soreness disappeared in a few days.

The second day, I received my first "food" at lunch time: chicken broth, apple juice, Jell-O, and tea. I didn't eat the Jell-O, wondering why they'd given it to me. Diabetics don't eat Jell-O; it's mostly sugar. The supper menu was a repeat of the noon meal, except it was beef broth, cranberry juice, Jell-O, and tea. This time I said, "I'm on a diabetic diet. Why are you giving me Jell-O?" The nurse quickly exchanged it for a dish of dietetic Jell-O, which I ate, although hospital Jell-O is more like rubber than food.

On Wednesday, I noticed swelling on my left arm where the IV was inserted. I mentioned it to a nurse, hoping the IV would be taken out permanently. My roommate's IV had already been removed, but they insisted on putting mine back in, but on the other hand, on the *top* of the hand—not an easy insertion and very uncomfortable because of the lack of flesh there. I hated it instantly. Wanting to be rid of it, I promised to drink all the liquids necessary to flush out my system, if only I could do without that painful IV. But the nurse wouldn't remove it. Dr. Lance called at six o'clock, explaining, "You need the IV because you're still running a slight fever. We have to be able to administer antibiotics quickly." *Why couldn't the nurse have explained that to me*, I wondered, *I would have accepted that explanation.*

The same day, I complained, "How can I get well and get rid of this IV if you don't give me any solid food?" Finally, a regular meal arrived for supper. I decided it paid to complain, just a little.

On Thursday, my fever was down. A nurse removed the hated IV from the top of my hand. Later, I learned Bud had told the desk nurse he felt my mental attitude was more important than having the IV. Whether that was the reason she removed it, I didn't know, but I didn't care. It was out.

Dr. Lewis removed the metal staples that held the incision together and put reinforced cellophane tape in their place. I looked like I was being held together with strapping tape. He said, "That will come off by itself in two weeks. You can shower with it on."

Dr. Lance came after lunch to give me the good news. "You can go home on Saturday, even if you're still running a low-grade fever. We would only keep you longer if your temperature should rise dangerously high. The pathologist's report showed everything to be benign."

Daily, I marveled at the small amount of pain I felt, compared to the pain I'd had before surgery. Satisfied with my progress, Dr. Lance said he planned to reduce my pain medication.

That afternoon, a nurse came to give me a hormone shot. Dr. Lance said I'd been given a hormone shot in surgery, however, so I refused it. Since I hadn't signed a release form for the shot before surgery, I signed it now. But we were never completely certain if I had gotten the hormone shot or not.

Friday, I walked down the hallway and had my first shower following surgery. I washed my hair and changed into my own comfortable pajamas. Mary, my best friend and neighbor, was waiting in my room when I returned. We visited until lunchtime.

I had a lot of company, including the visitation pastor from church. I wished the visits were spaced closer together or farther apart so I could nap longer. I took the pain pills only at night to help me sleep. I felt weak as a kitten. The nurses encouraged me to walk, walk, walk. I wondered if they knew how many trips I made to the bathroom each day now that the catheter had been removed. I tried to drink three thirty-ounce pitchers of water every day. I didn't want to risk getting a kidney infection and having the catheter or IV reinserted.

Intending to catch up on my reading, I had brought several books and magazines to the hospital with me. But when I tried to read, the words danced on the page. I kept losing my place. Finally, in frustration, I gave up reading. I decided it must be the pain medication. I was too doped up to read.

Saturday finally came— release day. I just wanted to go home. I couldn't bear to lie in bed another hour. I got up and sat in the easy chair next to my bed, behind the curtain that divided the beds. My arthritic back ached from too much time lying in bed. I started to read one of the books I'd brought with me, *I Ain't Well—But I Sure Am Better*[9] by Jess Lair.

When the nurse came to take my temperature and blood pressure, she couldn't find me. "Here I am." I spoke from behind the drawn curtain. I guess she thought I should be in bed. My temperature held at 99.6 degrees Fahrenheit, only slightly above normal. My blood pressure was 100/60—low but normal for me, especially in the morning.

Dr. Lance arrived shortly after lunch to discharge me. He wrote prescriptions for antibiotics, iron tablets, sleeping pills, pain pills, and hormone pills. "You're still running a slight temperature. I don't want to take a chance with infection," he said. "Otherwise, I wouldn't prescribe the antibiotic. Until I see you again in a couple of weeks, you shouldn't plan to do much more than what you're doing right now." Practically nothing! "Let your body be your guide."

I questioned him about the prescription for iron tablets. "That's what got me into this mess in the first place," I said.

"You need these iron tablets," he explained, "I saw this iron pouring out of your body. You should only have to take them for a few weeks." While I had lost some blood during surgery, it wasn't enough to require a blood transfusion.

I felt good. I wanted to stay up forever. I was so tired of lying in bed. I phoned Bud to come to the hospital to get me. Then I dressed in street clothes.

---

[9] Jess Lair, PhD. *I Ain't Well—But I Sure Am Better* (New York: Fawcett Crest Books, 1975).

As we checked out with my bag of unread books and magazines, one of the nurses commented, "I always get a chuckle out of all the literature people bring with them, thinking they'll have a chance to read. I know they won't feel like reading any of it."

I laughed. "Why didn't you tell me that before? I could have sent these books home with my husband yesterday."

As the nurse wheeled me down to the hospital release area, Bud drove up in our pickup truck. He lifted a cement block out of the truck bed and set it down on the ground so I wouldn't have such a big step to get into the cab. He also brought extra blankets to pad the seat, even remembering a small pillow to hold over my incision. Many friends told me about their first painful, bumpy ride home, but mine was quite comfortable.

Not having a lot of pain now, I wondered if the severed abdominal nerves were a blessing in disguise. Was the numbness masking pain? Or was God answering my prayers for freedom from pain?

I decided God was answering my prayers.

CHAPTER 16

"THEY DON'T GIVE MEDALS FOR ENDURING PAIN"

Bud, in his caring concern, made arrangements with our neighbor Mary to fix my lunch each noon. I knew eating was essential if I wanted to recover quickly—and I certainly wanted to recover quickly. I also wanted to regain the ten pounds I'd lost during surgery.

The soups I'd made and frozen before surgery tasted extra good now—beef vegetable soup one day; chicken vegetable with noodles the next—a healthy combination of protein and vegetables. Bud would take a plastic container of soup out of the freezer the night before so it could defrost in the refrigerator.

Dr. Lance had cautioned me not to push any heavy doors. I assumed that also meant pulling them. Our upright freezer door, with its tight-fitting seal, intimidated me. I could manage the refrigerator door, removing the soup with one hand, while holding my incision with the other. I spooned the soup into a glass bowl and popped it into the microwave for three minutes.

I didn't really need Mary's help—and I told her so—but for the first week, she continued to come each noon. I valued her friendship. Mostly, I treasured our lunchtime conversations. She was an important link to the outside world for me. We humans are social creatures. I already was suffering withdrawal pains from being isolated from others. Many friends seemed afraid to stop and visit, fearing, they said, that it would tire me. Yet I craved visits and welcomed human contact.

Wednesday, April 21, 1982

It took four days at home before I learned to pace myself—the amount of time I could stay up and the amount of time I needed to be flat on my back in bed. When I first came home from the hospital, I was so anxious to be up and out of bed that I spent too much time upright. The first clue, besides pain and fatigue, was increased blood flow. Mini-pads no longer sufficed; I had to change to maxi-pads, both day and night.

When he released me Saturday, Dr. Lance said my hemoglobin was down to 10.6—the lowest, to my knowledge, that it had ever been. He gave me a prescription for iron capsules—iron in a liquid form. Three days later now, I feel peppier but am still walking slowly. Dr. Lance said I lost about a pint of blood on the operating table but not enough to warrant a transfusion. When I questioned him about taking iron, since it was the root of a lot of my previous problems, he said, "You need this iron. This is hemorrhagic loss. I saw this iron flowing out of your body." It was a very convincing argument.

He ordered a week's supply of a tetracycline antibiotic, since I'm allergic to penicillin, Tylenol 3 (with codeine) for pain, and sleeping pills. So far, I've only needed to take one pain pill a day, usually at bedtime, except on Sunday when I took two because I spent too much time sitting up. On Tuesday, I took none, finally having learned to spend more time flat on my back.

Tonight, Bud apologized in advance in case he gets "short-tempered"; the lack of sleep is getting to him. I can tell he is getting tired. He gets up at 6:00 a.m. to make sure I have showered; then he makes breakfast and takes Mitzi for a walk before he leaves for work. I expected him to get grouchy, but so far he's been pleasant and cheerful—an inspiration to me. I know I could get depressed really fast if he wasn't so upbeat and helpful. I'm not a good patient; I have no patience!

Bud made it clear that although he will be glad when I can start doing little things around the house, like washing dishes or walking the dog, he doesn't want me to rush into doing things that might retard my recovery.

Tomorrow his mother is coming to get our laundry. She said she'd wash the dishes too. We must have two or three days' worth stacked in the sink. The neighbors have been good about bringing food—it adds a little variety to the soups, chili, and spaghetti in our freezer.

We finally received a call from our senior pastor. He called tonight at 10:30 to ask how I was doing—a week and a half after my surgery. Bud and I were both exhausted. We had gone to bed at 9:00 p.m. and were sound asleep when he called. I was furious for his lack of consideration and timing. I don't call well people at 10:30 p.m. unless it is an emergency. I saw no pastoral concern in his call. Had he called that late on the night before my surgery, I might have given him credit for some caring concern but not when I was recently home, recovering from surgery. What was he thinking?

Later I learned he made the call while getting ready to go out of town for a convention the next morning—his last opportunity to get information before Sunday morning's service, when he made a big production of announcing that he had called me during the week and that I was progressing nicely.

Was it unrealistic of me to expect more ministry from my pastor than a late-night call a week and a half after surgery and a Sunday morning announcement in church when I couldn't even be there to hear it? I didn't think so.

Poor Samantha, our black cat, was out of food one day, but I couldn't even bend over to replenish her food dish. She came meowing into my bedroom. Afraid she might jump up and land on my incision, I moved over to the far edge of the bed, trying to coax her up on the other side. I wanted to know exactly where she'd land. But the extra two inches of foam height on the bed must have intimidated her because she didn't jump. Frequently, she'd curl up on the bedspread that hung over the edge of the bed and cascaded onto the floor, purring contentedly to let me know she was close by and sympathetic. The two-inch foam mattress felt so good when I sank into its softness. I was thankful Van had suggested it.

I slept most afternoons, amazed when I woke up and found I had napped. Usually, I didn't feel tired when I lay down. A few days after I got home the phone woke me at 2:30 p.m. By the time I got out of bed and slowly shuffled down the hallway, it had stopped ringing. I shuffled back to bed but couldn't fall asleep. I needed to tell my friends if they were going to call, they should let the phone ring at least ten times. Without outside phone contact, I felt I might go stir crazy, being cooped up in the house for who knew how long.

People get so polite when you're ill. They don't want to bother you. They don't want to tire you. *Bother me! Tire me!* I wanted to say. *I need your human contact. You're my only link to the outside world!*

I typed a long letter to my mother, telling her about the surgery. Dr. Lance said he would give me a copy of his surgery report and the pathologist's report on May 5, my next office visit. I knew I was not feeling well because I didn't even care if I saw the reports. My typing was terrible! Could it be caused by the pain medicine, or had I gotten so rusty after only a week or two without practice? (It was the pain medicine.)

I questioned whether I would ever walk upright again without holding my incision. I felt like the pictures I'd seen of Cro-Magnon man.

Saturday, April 24, 1982

It's been a whole week since I came home from the hospital. When I left the hospital, I asked Dr. Lance if I could take a bath instead of a shower. He said I could, but Bud pointed out it might be harder to get out of the bathtub; plus, I might be more likely to slip getting in and out of the tub. The shower had no high sides to step over; I didn't want to accidentally pull something.

My daily shower is a high point of the day. The water streams onto my aching back muscles and over my body, rejuvenating me. The pulsating shower head gives a special massage to each little blood vessel, telling them to get moving and heal my body. Too much time flat on my back makes my arthritic back muscles ache, yet for every hour I'm up, I find I must spend at least one or two hours flat on my back. My first day home, I wanted to spend the entire recuperative period sitting up, reading, but my body revolted. Instead of standing tall when I walk, I find myself hunching over, especially when I don't get enough rest.

My body tells me that it hurts inside; I need to take the stress off my internal organs. Only bed rest helps. At other times, if I try to lengthen my "upright hours," my organs feel like they have shifted and are lying in a heap at the bottom of my abdomen. Your body is telling you to get into a prone position—I need to keep reminding myself of that. I've learned to read lying down.

Newspapers are the only thing I can't manage flat on my back. Sitting up, I find, is more tolerable if I can elevate my feet.

Relaxation and healing seem to go hand in hand. Although I didn't want to take any more pain pills than necessary, I found that not taking them when in extreme pain was foolish. If my muscles are all tensed up, they don't heal as quickly.

I've never been a day sleeper—sunshine in my window usually keeps me awake—but not this week. Sleep has a powerful curative effect. Even though I sleep several hours during the day, by eight o'clock at night, I long for bed again, often reading from my Bible for a half hour before taking my sleeping pill. Bible reading helps to relax me.

The cellophane tape across my incision loosened a little after each shower. Two weeks after surgery, my external incision looked healed—a thin red line. I marveled at the neat, straight line and remembered my words to Bud about Dr. Lance: "He'll have steady hands." The incision attested to my faith in my doctor's surgical abilities.

Mary commented that I was walking more upright. Sometimes I even forgot to hold my incision when I walked, but I didn't trust my body yet.

As my morning energy increased, I tried to plan projects for myself early in the day—letters and thank-you notes to write. It gave me something to do, a purpose for being. Having a project every day seemed important. During my recovery period, depression took a massive bite out of my mental resources. I wondered if that were true after all surgeries.

I relied heavily on my pain medications and sleeping pills. Asleep and relaxed, my body could heal itself; awake and agitated, I imagined my body was not healing. *Relax* was my mantra. *Get your body to relax.* Perhaps some people can relax without the aid of sleeping pills and pain meds, but I couldn't. When I didn't use the meds, I couldn't sleep. My body shifted constantly, trying to find a comfortable position. Finally, I concluded, *I'm not going to get hooked in a week.* Dr. Lance had advised me to take all my pain meds. "They don't give medals for enduring pain," he advised.

Because of the extensive surgery to my bladder and left kidney area, I knew the importance of keeping my urinary tract flushed out. "Drink!" they constantly reminded me at the hospital. At home, I tried to drink a glass of water every hour. Some days I drank more, some days less, but I usually drank my quota of eight glasses a day. I was more thirsty than usual and wondered if a low-grade fever contributed to my thirst. Fever was another reason to keep my body hydrated.

When urinating stopped hurting so much, I knew I was healing. Van said Dr. Lance said he had cut a lot of endometriosis off the bladder, and although he hadn't punctured the bladder, he had come close a few times.

But some days were still worse than others. I don't know why; my routine didn't vary. Some days were more pain-free, while other days I thought all my insides were going to slide out. Urinating and bowel movements were especially traumatic. I needed both bran flakes and stool softeners. I likened delivering a hard stool to delivering a "dry birth."

It portended to be a long, slow recovery.

CHAPTER 17

THE FEAR OF NOT KNOWING

Wednesday, April 28, 1982

It's been two and a half weeks since my surgery. For the first time this morning, I awoke feeling that I was starting to heal. Yesterday my body hurt constantly—all of it internal. Not a terrible pain, more like a constant stitch in my side, except it was in the abdomen. Two spots ached on each side of the navel. I imagined that's where the fallopian tubes had been glued to the bowel with endometriosis; now I experienced "ghost pain" from organs no longer there.

My incision is healing and growing thicker. It's a blessing to finally be able to walk down the hallway without having to hold my belly or feel that the slightest little jar to my body will crack it open like an egg.

The fever also seems to have broken. For the first time last night, my temperature was normal at bedtime. Finally, I can sleep without cushioning my incision with a pillow. The pillow, I feared, might become a permanent nighttime appendage.

Yesterday, I peeled off most of the filament tape covering my incision. It came off easily. Later I wondered, *Should I have removed it?* Only a few short pieces hold the incision together. My internal organs feel like they still need extra tape support. I found a roll of 3M surgical tape and taped across the incision. It helped momentarily, but being only paper tape, it didn't stay on very long.

Last Monday, I called Dr. Lance's office, asking if I could start wearing a panty girdle. I thought it would help support my internal organs. But the nurse advised against wearing a girdle until Dr. Lance checked the incision. My stomach still feels tender to touch, but if I rest a lot, it is pain-free.

I queried Dr. Lance's nurse about walking around the block; I miss my morning walks with Mitzi. I also asked if I could start helping around the house—doing dishes and other small chores. The monotony of doing nothing is driving me crazy. *I'll never, ever complain about doing dishes again,* I vowed to myself.

"You can do some small chores if you don't stand too long," the nurse instructed. A diplomatic no, I thought. I can wait. My appointment with Dr. Lance is a week away.

With nothing to do but contemplate the affairs of the world and my church, my thoughts turned to the similarities between the priorities of my holistic practitioners and the recent priorities of my church pastors.

Doctors Jim and Mary Berry were so involved with lecturing and spreading their perverted "gospel" for the American Holistic Medical Association, hoping to further the cause of their movement, that neither doctor adequately supervised their medical practice, which was now being run almost entirely by poorly trained nurse practitioners and doctor's assistants, who were dispensing much medical misinformation. Real problems were not addressed or treated, perhaps because these medical amateurs were unable to recognize real problems.

Likewise, my pastor, in an effort to become a powerful spiritual leader, busily ran from workshop to symposium, supposedly to sharpen his leadership skills in order to dispense pastoral wisdom, but he left sadly little time in his day to minister to the needs of his congregation—the people who, after all, paid his salary.

I drafted a letter to the church council, stating that I felt the church had grown too big to care about its individual members.

When my friend Irene stopped for coffee that afternoon, I shared my letter with her. She and her husband had recently left our church after consulting with the senior pastor for help with a personal problem. "Three times we asked for help," she said, "and three times he promised he *would* help. But he did nothing."

In the ensuing months, I heard more reports of congregational members who received neither pastoral visits nor spiritual counseling when faced with major surgery or other problems. The leadership workshops had not improved the caring ministry.

I seriously questioned why our church hired pastors at all—it should be for reasons other than administering the church's budget and social programs or preaching a sermon on Sunday morning. I likened going to church only for a Sunday morning service like going to a doctor only for his comforting bedside manner. That should *not* be the only reason for attending church. You go to a doctor for sound medical advice and knowledge. Likewise, a pastor should dispense spiritual direction and comfort.

I didn't want to leave my church. My Christian friends and supporters were in that church. If the pastor was the problem; that issue needed to be confronted.

In the past, I had written letters to our senior pastor, outlining problems I felt were developing in the church. I never received a response, not even an acknowledgment that the letter was received. This time, I wrote directly to the council president. He at least acknowledged receiving my letter.

Friday, April 30, 1982
No overnight bleeding last night. I'm hopeful that I'm finally healing inside. Today, I took my first walk outside, around the backyard, inspecting the tomatoes I'd planted before my surgery. How green and healthy everything looked. It felt so good to be outside again in God's green creation. I walked slowly around the grassy area twice.

This afternoon, while looking through old Arcadia Clinic medical bills, I noticed that when I suffered severe abdominal cramping in June 1979, Betty had written under diagnoses: "possible ovarian cyst? possible endometriosis?" Yet she never suggested that this could be a serious condition or that I should consult a gynecologist for further evaluation. As I looked further back in my file, Dr. Jim had diagnosed "anemia, iron deficiency" on one medical bill and "anemia, normocytic" on another. By now I knew the normocytic anemias were *not* caused by iron deficiency, yet he continued to treat me exclusively for iron deficiency.

A recent local newspaper article about endometriosis stated that early cases could be "burned out" with a new drug, Danazol, a synthetic hormone that created a pseudomenopause. The drug should be used for nine months. If adhesions blocked the fallopian tubes (as they did in my case), microsurgery could be performed to remove the obstruction. Fertility, in some cases, could be restored.

Bud and I read the article with distress. I was enraged. Dr. Jim never suggested that this type of obstruction could be the cause my infertility—or that it could be *corrected*.

Years later, Betty revealed Dr. Jim had suspected endometriosis as far back as 1973—about the same time he began treating me for anemia.

Sunday, May 2, 1982

Bud drove me to the store yesterday to buy fresh fruits and vegetables. Although walking in the store didn't bother me, I hurt later. The trip involved a lot of standing—waiting in line. Standing tired me more than walking. I finally asked Bud to check out the produce while I found a chair and sat down. My whole back and abdomen hurt, from my lungs and kidneys downward, including my legs. Then I remembered the nurse's cautioning, "Don't stand too long."

Always in the back of my mind lay the fear: Did I overdo? Did I accidentally tear loose some internal stitching? Did I permanently damage my internal repair work? And yet, I remembered Dr. Lance encouraging mild exercise—how much milder could I get than walking short distances?

Yesterday I took my first tub bath since surgery. Had I stretched my stomach muscles attempting to get settled into the tub without falling? Dr. Lance said I could take tub baths. He wouldn't have allowed it if he thought I would hurt myself. Fear—the unresolved stress of not knowing. *Relax*, I ordered myself—the secret to healing is to *relax*.

By nightfall, my incision appeared to be inverting, giving me an uneasy feeling that it could be sucked inward and expelled out with bladder and bowel movements. Was my body being turned inside out? Logically, I knew the impossibility of such a thing happening. But humanly, I worried.

Petting Samantha, our aged cat, was as relaxing as taking a tranquilizer. When I crawled into bed after breakfast, Sam came up to lie beside me. Bud had moved a hassock close to the bed so she could easily get onto the bed.

Sam seemed to understand the need to avoid jarring my body. She carefully walked onto the bed, gently lying down beside me, careful not to step on my body or to press too firmly against my abdomen as she often had in the past when, to her, closeness connoted affection. She lay next to me, near my waist, close enough that I could reach my hand down to stroke her body, softly, gently. She purred and I petted. It was a relaxing combination for both of us.

But just to be safe, I always put a pillow across my incision, in case she decided to exit the bed via my midsection, her usual route of departure before my surgery.

Months later, I realized that while Sam was comforting me, I also comforted her—a mutual sharing of suffering. In November while I improved, Sam, at age seventeen, died from cirrhosis of the liver, a common ailment in older cats.

CHAPTER 18

"THE BATTLE HAS ONLY BEGUN ..."

On May 5, my first visit with Dr. Lance three and a half weeks after being released from the hospital, I had another page of questions to ask.

Because my appointment was at 4:15 p.m., I spent most of the day lying on my back, resting my abdominal muscles.

Dr. Lance handed me his surgery report and the pathologist's report when we arrived. Then he checked my incision.

"The scar is healing fine," he reported. He didn't do an internal pelvic exam. "You can start driving if you feel like it." I really didn't feel like driving yet, but was glad to know I could if I wanted to.

"Tell me about the surgery again," I said. "Just what did you do? I was so drugged when you explained it the first time, I'm not sure I understood all you said."

Once again, he patiently repeated the information he'd given me in the hospital about the chocolate cyst and how it ruptured when they removed it, but that they had been prepared for this to happen.

I also wondered, *How close did I come to having the inflamed cyst burst when intense pain drove me to the emergency department in December?*

"Yours was an *endometrioma,*" Dr. Lance said, "an infectious cyst that was securely pasted onto the left pelvic side wall and ureter, caused by the endometriosis. Because of the extensive adhesions and the proximity of the cyst to the ureter, a small portion of the left ovary had to be left attached to the ureter. We didn't want to risk damaging the ureter by removing all of it. This could still cause future problems—even grow another cyst—but the chances of that happening are less than 2 percent. There also is a possibility of adhesions or scar tissue forming from the surgery, and the endometriosis could return because of the remaining piece of ovary." But he considered both of these possibilities slight (and nothing ever grew back).

"Why didn't you transfuse?" I asked.

"You hadn't lost that much blood."

"Did you consult with Dr. Fields about my low blood count?"

"No, the only time I saw Dr. Fields was when we passed in the hospital hallway and said, 'hi'."

It brightened my day to know Dr. Fields had come to the hospital to check on me out of concern, rather than in an official capacity. Finally, I'd found a caring doctor I could trust.

"You said the ultrasound showed hard and soft masses," I said. "What caused the hard masses?"

"Probably the adhesions," he replied. Adhesions, I learned later, show up on x-rays as calcium deposits.

"Did you ever get my reports from Arcadia Clinic?" I asked.

"So far, no, but I didn't feel I needed them," he responded.

To me, that wasn't the point. I had asked that the reports be sent to him a month ago, and he still had not received them. What if he *had* needed them? It was just another example of holistic medicine's slipshod practices with patient care.

I asked if he could tell how much longer it might have been before I would have had permanent kidney or bowel damage, but Dr. Lance did not want to speculate.

"Do you think I have the basis for a medical malpractice suit?"

He did not encourage this, explaining, "With endometriosis, it would be difficult to prove a time frame." Still, he felt Arcadia Clinic had been remiss if they suspected a cyst and/or endometriosis two years ago and did not refer me to a gynecological specialist for a more accurate diagnosis.

I thought again of Betty's saying, *"You don't want to have surgery, do you?"*

"Were you ever seen by a doctor about this diagnosis?" Dr. Lance asked.

"No. Betty, the nurse practitioner, was my only 'doctor' for the past several years. Dr. Berry told me she was trained to handle female problems. He implied she was only a few courses short of becoming a gynecologist." Now I knew that was not true.

Over the past few weeks of my recovery, I'd requested literature from the Arizona Nurses Association, specifically asking about nurse practitioners: What were they allowed to do and *not* allowed to do? Once I read their literature, I had a better understanding about what nurse practitioners were *not* permitted to do. For one thing, they were not allowed to write prescriptions.

"Even if I don't file a medical malpractice suit," I said, "I know to whom I should complain about my treatment. I intend to do something. Not once did Betty even suggest that infection and inflammation could be associated with endometriosis or that scar tissue could affect the surrounding organs, even though she thought I probably had endometriosis."

Suddenly angered again by this thought, I questioned: What did I, a lay person, know about this disease? She was the medical person who was supposed to be taking care of me.

"She always assured me that once I finished menopause, the endometriosis and its accompanying pain would disappear," I told Dr. Lance. "She implied that surgery was an unnecessary procedure." Rage flooded my soul, directed both at Betty and holistic medicine in general. Before I would have reached menopause, I likely would have died from peritonitis.

"One of the big problems with paramedic-type people," Dr. Lance suggested, "is getting them to refer patients to specialists when they are stumped." Then he said, "You probably will have pain for another month. Continue to take the pain pills as you need them."

"I have not taken any pain pills or sleeping tablets for the past week, not since April 28. I find I can best control the pain by lying down. Before that, I took the pain pills mostly at bedtime, as a relaxant. For me, pain pills worked better than sleeping pills."

Dr. Lance opened one of his medical books to show us pictures of endometriosis—it looked like the tissue of a severe burn victim. "Yours was one of the worst, most extensive cases, I'd ever seen."

Of course it was—it had been neglected for years. Scar tissue had been formed by the years of "burned out" endometriosis as my body's natural antibodies fought to control it. The edges of the scar tissue in the picture looked like tentacles as it grabbed and attached itself to the nearby abdominal organs, pulling them out of place and binding them together.

"Do you have any limitations for me?" I asked as we prepared to leave.

"Let your body be your guide," he answered.

Irene's husband, Johnnie, had prepared a delicious steak dinner for us. *Good red meat to restore my hemoglobin*, I thought, but I quickly tired, worn out from being up too long. We apologized and left shortly after eating.

The next day, May 6, I called Arcadia Clinic, demanding to know why my medical reports had not been sent to Dr. Lance. I requested that they be sent immediately. The desk girl replied that a notation in my file indicated they were sent on March 30.

"As of yesterday afternoon," I said, "they had not been received in Dr. Lance's office. Please send them again."

"Today is Betty's day off," she said, "but I'll send them this afternoon." I wondered if any pertinent information remained in my folder or if it had all been destroyed after my first call to Betty in which I informed her of her incompetence. Even after this call, Dr. Lance never received my files.

I had asked Dr. Lance if I could wear a panty girdle. He said I could, but he didn't think I would want to. After putting on a pair of tight Levi jeans, I agreed with him. I walked Mitzi to the corner of our block and back again. Afterward, I slipped into loose-fitting slacks. Following our walk, I noticed discharge again. More activity, more discharge. Would it ever stop?

It had been three weeks since my surgery. I finally felt strong enough to get dressed every day, but I still lay down during the day, fully clothed. I spent most of the time reading.

Sunday, May 9, 1982

It's been a month since my surgery, and I still have good days and bad days. Yesterday was not a good day. I want to help more with the household chores, so decided to wash several days of accumulated dirty dishes while Bud dried. I didn't even get finished when I had to quit to lie down. Standing in one spot seems to strain the abdominal muscles more than walking.

Wednesday, May 12, 1982

Life is full of small victories these days. Not only am I getting dressed every day, but I'm taking Mitzi for a walk—just to the end of the block and back, down the alley, a block-long round trip.

Marilyn, the president of our church's women's group, convinced me to attend a brainstorming meeting today. She thinks I need to get out of the house for a while and volunteered to pick me up, although it is quite a distance out of her way. I thought I needed to get out too, so I went. *It was a mistake.* The meeting started at 9:30 a.m. and lasted until 2:00 p.m.—about two hours too long for my abdominal muscles without bed rest. And it extended past my lunchtime; I felt hypoglycemic. Marilyn generously shared her cheese, crackers, and apple slices with me. Afterward, I wondered if it would have been smarter to hold the meeting in my unkempt house, where I could have lain down when tired and eaten when hungry.

On the way home, I asked Marilyn to drive me to a nearby print shop so I could make copies of the finished June district newsletter, *The Communicator.* Thankfully, I had this creative activity to work on while confined. It helped keep me sane. Next day Bud mailed the pages for me.

In response to the letter I wrote to the church council president, our church secretary called today. She set up an appointment for the assistant pastor to visit tomorrow. I need to do some heavy praying tonight so I know what to discuss with him. I have a lot of bitterness to resolve.

I feel depressed today and wonder if it is the aftereffects of losing my reproductive organs or if my hormones are out of balance—or both. I called Dr. Lance, asking if I should take the hormones for twenty-five days, then off for five days, the same as birth control pills. He answered, "yes". I am taking 0.125 milligram of estrogen, half of what I was taking under Betty's care before surgery.

To a person like me, who has enjoyed good health most of her life, it is a terrible revelation to realize that humanly, I am subject to the same bodily frailties as everyone else. My holistic doctors had thoroughly brainwashed me to believe if I followed their healthy practices, I would *never* get sick.

Tonight I carefully threaded my way through a crowded grocery store, fearing someone would accidentally bump my incision. I vowed that in the future, I would try to be more understanding of the frailties of older and ill persons but then wondered how soon I would forget that resolve, when I wasn't hurting anymore. Perhaps God allows illness sometimes to sharpen our senses toward other people.

Thursday, May 13, 1982

I can't seem to stop crying today. Is my body trying to adjust to the artificial hormones? Or are the natural hormones still trying to dissipate from my body? Or is it from something entirely different? Maybe it has nothing to do with my organs at all. Maybe it is connected to other losses—the loss of a doctor I trusted. The loss of a church I revered. The loss of a friend I valued. The loss of children we'll never have.

I am tempted to cancel my appointment with Pastor Walker this afternoon, but that would only be running away

from the problem or denying that a problem exists. If I
refuse to confront this problem, I would be no better than
Tim Rogers, our senior pastor. We can't run away from our
problems forever—but we do try at times.

I blubbered my way through Pastor Walker's visit. I didn't intend to
cry, but I couldn't stop. I asked point-blank why I hadn't been contacted
before surgery to see if I needed spiritual counseling or prayer. He said
he didn't know about my surgery until Tuesday, the day after surgery,
when Pastor Rogers told him I should be visited.

"I don't blame you," I said, "I blame Pastor Rogers. On Palm
Sunday, he knew about my surgery, even commented about members
going in for surgery around Easter. But he chose to do nothing about it.
Was I supposed to make an appointment if I wanted a visit? Did I slip
up? Did I not tell the right people? Who are we supposed to contact?
Your secretary knew. Didn't she tell you? Did she tell anyone? I thought
when a member of the office staff was told of an impending surgery, the
staff would know who to alert. Is there no organization in this church?"

"You should call the front desk and tell Joy," he answered quietly.

"And how are we, the parishioners, supposed to know that?" I
demanded. "I have never seen any instructions, any chain of command.
When I talk to someone in the office, I figure that person will know
whom should be told. Joy does not always answer the phone. If the
office staff doesn't know whom to tell, how am I supposed to know? My
doctor came to visit me the night before my surgery, concerned about
my physical and mental health, but my pastors were not concerned
about my spiritual health." There; I had voiced it.

"Furthermore," I prattled on, "Bud also feels upset that none of the
pastors gave either of us any kind of spiritual support. When his dad
had open-heart surgery, our pastor at that time sat through the whole
operation with us. Bud's not a bit interested in this church anymore. He
says all they're interested in is whether or not we pay our pledge on time.
If the church doesn't support us, why should we support the church? If
he wants to leave and go to a different church, I'll have to go with him.

I need a church home, whether it's Church of the Valley or not. But *I* don't want to change churches," I said, sobbing. "All my friends are here. Why should I have to change churches?"

Pastor Walker listened sympathetically, apologizing for the church's neglect. But he did not encourage us to stay. Instead, he said, "Whatever you decide, I hope you will not give up going to church entirely."

"I will never give up going to church," I said.

"Would you like communion?" he asked.

"No," I replied, "I can't take communion feeling like this." He said he understood.

Friday, May 14, 1982

Dorothy Dorring, one of the older women in my prayer circle, stopped to visit this afternoon, bringing some religious tapes. We had a long talk, including my feelings about the uncaring ministry of the church. Later, I wondered if she had come as a member of my prayer circle, as a Christian friend, or as a representative of the Church Council—or all three. I didn't care. A truly spiritual person, Dorothy would not misinterpret my concerns.

I told her about my premonitions—the one that warned I had only three years to live—and the latest that the cancer was not in my ovaries.

The thought occurred to me that the Good Friday premonition that the cancer was not in my body might have been God's way of telling me that the cancer was *in the church*. I didn't mention that thought to Dorothy. Instead, I shared my concerns about the ache in my left shin.

"I have to get it all checked out," I told her.

While we talked, a refrain from the movie soundtrack *The Alamo* raced through my mind, "You think, sir, the battle is over . . . the battle has only begun. ..."

CHAPTER 19

SPIRALING DOWN INTO DEPRESSION

On Friday I thought I was getting better. I felt stronger and had energy into the evening. I was able to stand up straighter. I didn't have the feelings of weepiness. Friday was the first of the five days off the hormones—the time of the month I should be menstruating. Is this weepiness my body's crying for the loss of this function? I never expected to feel sad to see the end of my menstrual cycles.

My body feels like it is healing in layers. Often I feel better over the weekends, as if I have completed a layer of healing. During the week, I feel punk again. Perhaps I overdo when I'm feeling better. Today, Sunday, May 16, I feel fatigued; my pelvic bones ache. My hips are still sore from all the pain shots after surgery.

I washed three days' worth of dirty dishes, sitting down between stretches so I wouldn't get too tired. It took almost two hours and wore me out so much that I spent the rest of the afternoon in bed.

For the first time this morning, I drove myself to the grocery store. Although I didn't notice any internal pulling, I felt shaky and unsure of my driving. It's been five weeks since my surgery. I bought two six-packs of soda and carried them into the house. Afterward, I noticed more pelvic pain and wondered if they were too heavy for me to be carrying so soon.

Every day, I massage my right hip and thigh. Sometimes I think the feeling is returning. Other times, it feels as numb as ever.

Tuesday, May 18, 1982

I am really hurting today—a dull ache on the left side where I imagine the left ovary was located. The pain reminds me of the pain I had before surgery. Is it caused by my driving yesterday, my carrying the two six-packs of soda, or intestinal gas from the soda I drank last night? When I rested this afternoon, it subsided briefly but returned in the evening, forcing me to bed early. Am I pushing *too hard* to do things and not lying down often enough?

The spotting has almost completely stopped. I expected it to be stopped long before now—a five-week-long menstrual period. I hope it means the healing is almost complete; that this pain won't last forever.

Crowds are disconcerting, especially crowds of friends. Growing up on a farm as the only girl between two brothers, I was a loner. Now I prefer single-person visits from a few close friends or neighbors who remain constant and nonjudgmental during this ordeal with depression.

My first venture into group social activities was a women's church meeting. I'd talked so much about my surgery that I didn't want to hear one more question about it; thus, I was reluctant to face a barrage of comments from acquaintances who hadn't yet asked the polite questions, such as "How are you doing?" When the meeting date finally arrived, I was glad for an excuse to come late. One of our members, whose husband was having health problems, asked me to pick her up but said she couldn't leave until his needs were met.

I'm forever grateful to the women who simply hugged me and said, "It's so nice to have you back." This left me free to reply, "It's good to be back" and really mean it.

But even though I was glad to be there, I was already looking ahead to next month's meeting with dread, glad that summer meetings were discontinued. Next month's June meeting would be the last time I'd have to face this crowd of friends until fall. By fall, I hoped my mental outlook would be improved.

Tuesday, May 18, 1982, later

I am reading several chapters in my Bible every night before turning out the light. It seems to help block the pain momentarily. I started reading the Gospels, then the Book of Psalms, and now I'm into Paul's letters.

I haven't been teary for several days. I've been off estrogen for five days, but tonight starts a new cycle.

Wednesday, May 19, 1982

I really hurt today so decided not to drive for a while. It's not worth the pain. I finally took a pain pill. I still feel like I'm healing in layers. I wonder how many more layers I have to go.

I'm teary again today. Is it from frustration or from being back on the estrogen?

Thursday, May 20, 1982

I'm glad Dr. Lance warned that I might still need pain pills. I'm taking both pain pills and sleeping pills at night again. I thought I was finished spotting, but this morning I noticed a thick, pus-like discharge. I hope I'm into the last stages of healing. I'm so weary of this long process.

I forgot the stool softener last night. No bowel movement today. The ache wraps around my whole body, traveling halfway down my legs. Did I have this surgery—and still not solve the problem?

Pastor Borglund, the visitation pastor, stopped to visit me this afternoon. We had a long talk. He apologized, saying he was the pastor who *should have* visited me before surgery, but he was on vacation. I expressed my misgivings about Pastor Rogers's ability to shepherd our congregation.

"When you know what is right to do, and don't do it," I said, paraphrasing scripture, "you are still accountable to God." I thought Pastor Rogers had a lot of accounting to do.

I related the story about the neighbors we had brought into the church through the neighborhood shepherding program—how they had asked Pastor Rogers for help with counseling for their daughter and son-in-law who, they felt, were falling away from church. Three times they asked for Pastor Rogers's help. Each time he said he would talk to the young couple, but he never did. Our friends left the church.

"Why should we witness and get people involved in our church," I asked, "only to have the pastor drive them away with disinterest? The pastors have plenty of time to attend out-of-town conferences and meetings that are supposed to make them better pastors, but they don't have time to minister to their own members. Our church's priorities are in the wrong place."

He listened politely. Before leaving, he asked, "Would you like to have communion?"

"I've prayed about this a lot," I responded, "and I've asked God for a sign. When I get the sign, I will know what to do about my membership. Until then, I cannot take communion."

After Pastor Borglund left, I felt relief. I'd shared my concerns with everyone I thought could initiate change in the church. Now it was out of my hands.

Thursday, May 20, 1982, later

Tonight severe pain gripped me—it felt like it was in the bone instead of the abdomen. Why is new pain appearing now, five and a half weeks after surgery? It's a dull, throbbing, unrelenting pain in the bone. Is it cancer? Arthritis? Or what?

When Bud came home from work, I summarized my visit with Pastor Borglund. "He quoted a lot of Bible verses to me," I said, "and I quoted some back to him, including James 4:17. 'If you know what is right to do, and fail to do it, for you, it is sin.'" In a flash the thought occurred to me, *But isn't that just what* you're *doing?*

"I guess that verse applies to me just as much as it does to Pastor Rogers," I said. "If I don't forgive him, I'm no better than he is."

Friday, May 21, 1982

I called Dr. Lance for a renewal of my pain medication. He renewed it without question. The shooting pains in my left leg have spread to my right leg.

Dorothy Dorring, bless her heart, visited again, bringing some Bible studies. I returned the materials she left on her first visit. "The theology in the books you left," I explained, "is too deep for me to absorb right now. I need lighter stuff—music that I can listen to when I lie down in the afternoon."

We talked about my visit with Pastor Borglund. I mentioned being concerned that no one was ministering to Bud's spiritual needs. While both Pastors Walker and Borglund visited me, Bud had received no ministry. "No one except me is ministering to Bud," I said sadly.

After confiding these concerns to Dorothy, I felt more at peace, telling her, "It's out of my hands now. I have done all I can. I can do no more."

I felt I had reached the end of another healing layer. Tonight I didn't need a pain pill.

Friday night we began decorating the ballroom for Bud's parents' fiftieth wedding anniversary celebration. I didn't help; instead, I just sat and offered suggestions, hoping they were helpful. We didn't get back home until ten o'clock. I went straight to bed, exhausted, but awoke at 2:30 a.m. needing to empty my bladder. The pain was back. I took a pain pill. My bowels rumbled all night. I slept fitfully.

I'm still taking the daily iron capsule to build up my blood but forgot to take one at noon. The anniversary celebration lasted from two to four that Saturday. Besides not having my iron pill, I didn't get an afternoon nap and was exhausted when we returned home at six. Now I realized how much the iron tablets were helping. I took one and went to bed. Bud said I slept for two hours, awaking at eight.

"Perhaps we should go to church with your folks tomorrow, in honor of their fiftieth anniversary," I suggested when I woke up.

Bud was pleased. "Maybe this is your sign," he said. The issue, I finally realized, was not whether Pastor Rogers was a forgivable person but whether I was a forgiving person.

Sunday, May 23, 1982

I thought Pastor Rogers tried hard to make amends. He made a big production out of Bud's folks celebrating their fiftieth wedding anniversary—he even asked them to stand and be recognized during the church service.

In the afternoon, we drove to Tom and Van's for a small private family picnic with close relatives. I didn't do much except eat and sit—but even that was too much.

Tuesday, May 25 1982

I'm having trouble with constipation; the stool softeners are not working. Some days I don't even have a bowel movement. I finally called Dr. Lance. He suggested I come into his office tomorrow, before my six-week appointment with Dr. Fields.

I'm having so much pain lately. I was afraid I'd developed a hernia from carrying the two six-packs of soda. However, upon his examination, Dr. Lance found no indication of hernia. The groin pain, he suggested, was probably caused by the sigmoid bowel adjusting itself. When I told him my stools weren't soft anymore, he gave me samples of a stool softener with a laxative in it. "Keep your stools soft," he ordered.

"I noticed mild groin pain shortly after surgery when I used the bathroom. It seems like a cord or muscle has gotten stuck in the bend of my left thigh where it joins the body," I complained. At the time, I thought, *I hope the doctors didn't get the ureter stuck down in that crease.* "The ureter doesn't go down to that area, does it?" I had finally voiced my concern.

He replied that it did, but he didn't think it was the problem. "If the pain doesn't disappear in the next few months, we'll redo the kidney dye test."

"Could a muscle have gotten moved during surgery and is now

getting hung up when I bend my leg?" I queried. Because sitting required bending, it aggravated the groin pain.

"We didn't work with the muscles in that area," he reassured me. "Besides they are pretty firmly attached. But we worked on the pelvic bone under the muscles. The pain might be from a muscle strain." He suggested I apply a heating pad to the area for a few days.

When I visited Dr. Fields the next day, I asked if the chocolate cyst had been responsible for my anemia.

"Maybe part of it," he said, "but not all of it." He still thought a low hemoglobin count might be normal for me, that my bone marrow was just not producing red cells properly.

"You said before that my bone marrow was producing plenty of red cells," I reminded him.

"Yes," he agreed, "but not enough to replenish those being destroyed in your system. The hemoglobin count is still low at 12.2 but up almost two points in the six weeks since your surgery."

Apparently, this time the iron tablets were doing their job.

Our good neighbors and best friends, Mary and Marshall, put their house up for sale. We were not happy to see their For Sale sign, but we understood their reasons for wanting to move. Sandy, their youngest daughter, was still in high school, and our neighborhood high school was closing.

Friday, May 28, 1982

It's been almost seven weeks since my surgery. I expected to be back to normal after six weeks. Bone pain continues to plague me—the left pelvis, shin, and ankle. It's not severe pain but constant—and frustrating.

I'm anxious to do things. I want to be healed. I try to work on my book each day, knowing that I need to get into a routine, lest boredom drives me into a deep depression.

Today, I experienced some of the old lightheaded spaced-out feelings. I am not sleeping well. The laxative/stool softeners rumble nightly in my intestines.

Saturday, May 29, 1982

Today I feel like my old, bubbly, happy self again, which makes me think I've emerged from a period of depression. Yet I never consciously felt depressed. Maybe that is how depression creeps up on people.

Before Bud left for work, I asked him to take out the vacuum cleaner for me. While he was at work, I started vacuuming the living room—until I got a stitch in my side, where I imagined Dr. Lance had removed the appendix. *Maybe I shouldn't be using the vacuum cleaner so soon*, I thought—so I quit.

Sunday, May 30, 1982

I don't know what to think about my aches anymore. Today I have aching in the rib cage, spinal area, and lower back—all on the left side. Not intense and not constant, but I am just so tired of being sick.

Harriet loaned me a book, *Nineteen Steps Up the Mountain*,[10] the story of Dorothy and Bob DeBolt, who, in addition to raising their own children, took in fourteen handicapped children. I need that kind of inspirational reading right now.

Monday, May 31, 1982

After using the heating pad for several days, the groin pain finally released or relaxed. Perhaps the sigmoid bowel has unkinked. It seems that one side of my body goes through a healing process, then the other side—never both sides together.

Tuesday, June 1, 1982

Crowds are becoming a problem for me. Bud and I went to Fedmart's going-out-of-business sale yesterday. Overwhelming tiredness and dread smothered me with the

---

[10] Joseph P. Blank. *Nineteen Steps Up the Mountain* (Toronto, Ont.: Jove Books (Harcourt Brace). 1977).

thought of standing in a long check-out line—so much so that I didn't buy anything. On our way to the car, Bud met a postal friend and stopped to chat. I fidgeted, wanting to get out of the store and into the wide open spaces of the parking lot. Do I have agoraphobia? Fear of being in public or open places? Finally, I whispered to him, "I've got to get out of here." So he said good-bye and we left.

Already I'm considering not going to the June women's meeting at church this Thursday, although I know I should get out with people more. I wonder if I'm getting used to being confined to the house. Am I starting to enjoy the solitude? Is that healthy? Maybe I gadded too much before surgery, and now God wants me to take time for my writing. I don't feel tired in the morning when working on writing projects, but the thought of crowds panics me. Am I getting claustrophobia (fear of enclosed spaces) or agoraphobia?

Wednesday, June 2, 1982
I feel strong today. I drove to Dr. Lance's office for my first pelvic exam since the surgery. It's been seven and a half weeks.

"Your weight is a pound less than last week," the nurse commented.

"That's probably from the laxative Dr. Lance recommended." I laughed.

"Everything looks good. You're progressing normally," Dr. Lance said after the exam. "You still look a little swollen and inflamed on the left side where we had to scrape the bone. You are actually doing very well for the amount of surgery you had done."

Scraped the bone? That was the first I knew he had scraped the bone. No wonder the pain felt like bone pain. The healing is reaching down to the bone layer.

"Have you resumed intercourse yet?" he asked.

"No, we were waiting for permission. Is it okay?"

He said it was. He asked about the groin pain. I said it had relaxed on Monday. Whether from the heat or the laxatives, the pain was gone. "Take the stool softener now only as needed," he advised.

"Yesterday I noticed that some of the iron is being thrown overboard into my stools," I said, recognizing the familiar black streaks that indicated my body didn't need all the iron it was getting.

"That's a good sign. Your body is catching up on iron," he said. "Dr. Fields will follow up on your iron treatment."

I mentioned that my breasts were quite tender and that Dr. Fields had commented I already displayed some changes in the breast tissue. Dr. Lance reduced the estrogen dose from 1.25 milligrams to .0625 milligrams—a quarter of the 2.5 milligrams Betty had me taking before my surgery, an amount Dr. Lance had said was much too strong for my needs. I wondered if my holistic healers had been trying to *give* me breast cancer, along with everything else.

Dr. Lance found no sign of vaginal infection; the abdominal area was mostly pain-free to pressure, except for a few shooting pains, which he ascribed to scarring or healing still taking place in those areas.

He gave me permission to fly back for my niece Elaine's wedding in early July but cautioned, "Don't *you* carry any heavy bags. You won't damage yourself permanently anymore, but you might pull a muscle internally that could cause unnecessary pain. Are you having any discharge?"

"No bleeding, but I have a pus-like discharge."

"That should cease shortly," he reassured. I hoped so. After wearing a sanitary pad for seven and half weeks, I felt like I had returned to infancy—and diapers.

"Can I start taking walks again?" The wives of many of the men Bud worked with, who had had hysterectomies, resumed walking after the third week.

"No," he said emphatically. "It's not necessary. You're not overweight. And you don't need the exercise. Apparently, you are getting enough exercise. Just continue to do the same things you are doing now."

He didn't need to see me again for six months. "Come back around Christmas."

Dr. Lance said I had another month of healing ahead of me, but now I'm bothered by insomnia. I decided to use up the remaining sleeping pills.

I went to the church women's meeting the next day but didn't stay for the whole meeting. Florence, one of the women in my circle, called, asking if I could pick her up. Her husband, who is recovering from a stroke, had a therapist scheduled to come in, so she could get away for a few hours, but she couldn't leave until just before lunch. I welcomed the chance to go later. I wanted to go, but didn't want to stay a long time.

Crowds, even with familiar friends, still made me anxious. But I was glad to be able to help Florence. She needed to get out with people, too. She didn't drive, so her life was even more confined than mine, especially since her husband's stroke.

We both had a good time. I collected hugs, thankful no one mentioned my surgery. I didn't want to talk about it, now that I was on the road to recovery.

Friday, June 11, 1982

Today is my last day on estrogen before the five-days-off period. The past few nights I've felt intensely fatigued and went to bed at 8:30 instead of my usual ten o'clock. I'm feeling melancholy and teary again. Is it postsurgical depression and changes to my body? I'm having a hard time adjusting.

We finally had sex. I thought I was ready. Bud was so gentle and lovingly tried to make sure he didn't hurt me. But it was a big *nothing*! No pain. No pleasure! I felt numb inside. *Is this what they mean about feeling like "half a woman" after hysterectomy?* I wondered. My only consolation was that, for me, hysterectomy had not been an option; it had to be done to save my life. Still, I am filled with *rage* against Arcadia

Clinic and the holistic medical staff who let my condition deteriorate, necessitating such major surgery.

After bathing, I began to cry. I couldn't stop. Bud found me in the bedroom. I told him about my feelings of frustration and the meaninglessness of sex. I wanted him to know that if I was less than enthusiastic, it had nothing to do with my feelings toward him. I felt like I had been *spayed*. They neuter animals to curb their sex drive. Why don't doctors address that problem with women?

Whenever I begin to feel strong physically, the mental depression sets in. Or was the depression there all along, overshadowed by the physical pain? When you are physically ill, it is easy to blame the depression on physical causes, but as I grow stronger, the mental depression had to be faced as an entity unto itself. I needed to motivate myself to *do* things.

In an attempt to work my way out of the lethargy, I found it necessary to plan my day; to always have something to look forward to for the next day. Working on my book was part of the therapy, and editing and typing articles for *The Communicator* district newsletter gave me a creative boost. I forced myself to stick with a task until I had completed something—a chapter in my book or a page or two of the newsletter. My writing gave me pleasure and a reason to face each new day.

A few weeks before, in an attitude of love, Harriet Hammon mentioned she was concerned that I might be sinking into depression. Until her comment, I hadn't considered mental depression, but I found a copy of Leonard Cammer's book *Up from Depression*[11] in a used-book store. I bought the book. As I read it, I found my symptoms of depression more closely resembled a *reactive* (grief) depression than an *endogenous* (organic or physical) depression, such as would follow surgery or the manic-depressive symptoms that herald severe emotional problems. I wondered, what I could be grieving. Was it the loss of children we would never have?

---

[11] Leonard Cammer. *Up from Depression* (New York: Simon & Schuster Pocket Books, 1969).

Monday, June 14, 1982
It's been nine weeks since my surgery. I finally gathered enough nerve to put on a panty girdle. It felt okay. After buying a new box of panty liners, the discharge finally seems to be ceasing.

Wednesday, June 16, 1982
Abraham Lincoln once said, "Next to creating life, the greatest thing one can do is save a life." Since I could no longer "create life," I decided I would try to save lives.

I wrote a five-page letter to the Arizona Nurses Association, complaining about Arcadia Clinic's inadequate treatment in my case and Betty's incompetence as a licensed nurse practitioner. I sent a carbon copy of the letter to the Arizona Medical Association.

A few days later, I received a reply from the Arizona Nurses Association, stating they didn't feel they were the proper agency to handle my complaint. They requested that if I wished it to be forwarded to the Arizona State Board of Nursing, I should indicate that wish in writing. I responded that they had my permission to forward my complaint to the Arizona State Board of Nursing—and whoever else had jurisdiction over this type of complaint. They also forwarded a copy of my letter to the Arizona Board of Medical Examiners.

CHAPTER 20

OUT OF CONTROL

Friday, June 25, 1982

Tomorrow we leave for Elaine's wedding in Wisconsin. My body is again a battleground of unexplained aches and pains, shooting pains in the pelvic bone, sharp pains in the area where the bone marrow was extracted, followed by a quick, burning sensation, plus all the usual aches and pains in my left leg and rib cage. And my weight seems to be down slightly. I wonder why.

After two weeks visiting with my family in Wisconsin, I was glad to be home again in my own bed. What doctors described as an inner ear infection marred most of my Wisconsin visit. It started on Tuesday, the third day after our arrival—lightheadedness that proceeded to a dizzy, spinning sensation whenever I moved my head too quickly. I first noticed it when I awoke Tuesday morning and turned over in bed; the room went into a rapid spin. Nausea followed the dizziness and vomiting followed the nausea. After emptying my bowels, I felt some relief.

The clinic doctor we consulted diagnosed it as an inner ear infection, probably brought on by a sinus infection, compounded by the high altitude of flying, which, he said, drove the virus into the inner ear. I didn't understand why the condition hadn't shown up earlier instead of three days after flying. I couldn't recall ever suffering from a sinus infection in the past, before or after flying; although on occasion I had noticed some lightheadedness, which I associated with sinus congestion. As a precaution, now I always took an antihistamine before flying.

By the time I visited my mother's medical clinic, the vomiting had stopped and did not recur, but the nausea and dizziness persisted for most of the remaining two weeks, leaving me miserable. Once again, I experienced the old spaced-out feeling. My brain felt numb, like it was packed with cotton fuzz.

The clinic doctor prescribed Meclizine, an anti-vertigo drug, and told me to move slowly.

"You'll probably want to lie down the first day," he advised. Although I followed his advice at first, I felt less dizzy in an upright position. I practiced moving slowly to avoid jarring my head. The drug provided minimal relief, but as the symptoms persisted into the second week, I renewed the prescription and was able to attend my niece's wedding.

As I debated whether to risk flying back to Phoenix and reinfecting my inner ear, two days before our scheduled departure date the dizziness and nausea disappeared. In its place, a melancholia depression settled in. I was nearing the end of my twenty-five-day estrogen cycle again.

We arrived home on Saturday. After two weeks without sex, now I was sure that my body had had time to heal. I looked forward to making love with my husband and knew Bud was looking forward to it too. I was proud of him for his loving patience.

But sex produced pain. It felt like my vagina was too short. Naturally, the pain put a damper on any sexual pleasure. Was this to be the pattern of our future lovemaking? Pain? Always pain?

Bud, unaware of my immediate feelings, was more concerned about the numbness from the severed nerves that prevented me from experiencing sexual pleasure. He asked, "Did you feel anything?"

"Pain," I replied bitterly.

"At least you felt *something*." He sounded jubilant. That was the wrong reaction.

"Do you think that's going to make me more eager to have sex?" I asked, hurt by his response. A deep, overwhelming urge to cry bathed me with tears of frustration, but I didn't want him to see me cry. I didn't want him to know that his unfeeling remark had hurt as much as the act. I held back my tears as I hurried to shower.

In the shower, I discovered bright-red fresh blood. I was bleeding again. A flood of despair crept over me. Would the bleeding never end? It had been three months since my surgery. Would I never get well? Would I never heal?

A mini-pad was not enough. Again, I had to resort to maxi-pads and was thankful I still had a supply.

Bud had gone to the living room to watch TV, so I lay on the bed and cried into my pillow. I had lost the ability to cope with my feelings, both toward the hysterectomy and toward my husband. It was a short, body-wrenching release of emotion, but when I finished crying, I felt better and joined him in the living room.

I wore the maxi-pad all night. Next morning I was still bleeding—profusely. It was as if I had started my periods all over again. *I thought I was finished with periods*, I thought sorrowfully.

After church, Bud expressed frustration and guilt. "I blame myself," he said. "I should have been more gentle and careful."

"No one told us we had to take it easy *forever*," I replied, trying to make him feel better. "How were we to know? I should be healed by now. It's been three months. All the books I read said 'six to eight weeks.' Tomorrow, I'll make an appointment with Dr. Lance. He said I should come back if the pain persisted."

Even though it was Sunday afternoon, Bud went to the post office to work for a few hours. I was jealous of the time he spent at work. He seemed to escape to work more often because he didn't know how to react to my outbursts and silences. We were becoming strangers. I didn't understand my temperament either or how I should react. *He can escape to work*, I thought bitterly, *but I have to stay here and live with myself.*

While on vacation, I'd learned that one of my younger first cousins had SLE—systemic lupus erythematosus. One thing I didn't need to hear was that lupus existed in our family; it's a familial disease. Did I have lupus instead of arthritis when my doctor advised me to move to a warmer, dryer climate? My symptoms were not as severe as my cousin's, yet there were similarities. Could lupus be the reason for my slow healing?

Three months of being sick following surgery, preceded by a year of fatigue before that, had taken its toll on my patience. At times I felt myself drifting deeper and deeper into a pit of depression. Would I be sucked into the depths of insanity too?

The periods of melancholia would intensify and then subside. I found myself crying over the least little insignificant thing and didn't know why. They were not body-wracking sobs but weeping. The tears came and went. My nose would drip, and I would wipe it; the emotions were all just below the surface.

Other times, I felt like a volcano, ready to explode. I fought to suppress that feeling and maintain control of my body and emotions.

I imagined myself as a drowning person on a cork, bobbing up and down in the water. Just when I thought I was coming out of the depression, I sank down again, each time a little deeper than the last, fighting all the time to break through to the surface but never quite able to get my head above water.

When Bud came home from work, we went out for supper. The melancholy mood that had been building all day exhibited itself halfway through our meal. I began to weep. Tears streamed down my face, unchecked. I had lost the ability to control my emotions. I gazed into space, avoiding Bud's eyes, which I knew were watching me with questioning concern. I was afraid he'd ask, "What's the trouble?" And then I'd make a scene in the restaurant, blowing up and going stark raving berserk. Thankfully, he remained silent.

When we returned home, I felt I owed him an explanation. We were standing in the kitchen when I said, "I think I'm losing it." I waited for him to ask, "Losing what?" But he remained silent, so I continued.

"I feel like I'm drowning—like I'm sinking deeper and deeper into a depression that I'll never get out of." I was crying hysterically and was totally frustrated. I had reached an abyss. Was I on the brink of insanity?

Bud pulled me to his chest and held me close. "No, you aren't, Baby," he soothed. "I won't let you. Just let it all out."

I exploded in a burst of fury and shoved him away. Turning my back on him, I clenched my teeth and my fists and jumped up and down on the floor—totally out of control. I felt like a person possessed by a demon. I felt violent. I screamed at him, "Leave me alone. I *do* blame *you*!" I said, referring to his comment the previous night after we had sex.

I had heard of acts of violence committed under the guise of temporary insanity, and while I don't believe I could have gone against the strict, moral Christian code with which I had been brought up and physically harmed myself or Bud, in that instant of rage, I didn't know what I might be capable of doing. I was *afraid* of what I might be capable of doing. Yet I knew *what* I was doing— I just couldn't stop!

Although I never consciously considered suicide such as shooting myself, I had an uncontrollable urge to fling myself through a plate-glass window. I wished we were on the top floor of a twenty-story building so I could jump through the window and swan dive down to my death. I wanted to get away from *myself.* The story in Mark's Gospel about the demon-possessed swine plunging off a steep cliff to drown in the sea came to mind.

But I didn't want to jump through just any plate-glass window. Our arcadia door that opened into the backyard had a plate glass window. I didn't consider jumping through it. My rational mind told me that jumping through a ground-floor door or window would *not kill me,* but it might maim and slice up my body so badly that I'd have to go back to the hospital for more surgery. The *last* thing I wanted was more surgery. My world was shattering around me in huge, jagged pieces of broken dreams.

I clenched my fists in a concerted effort to regain control of the demon raging within my body. I wanted to prevent it from causing harm to me or anyone else. I knew I needed to get control of my emotions, yet I felt locked in a life-or-death struggle with my own body.

Later, I as I reflected on this incident, I wondered, *Was it a life-or-death struggle for my body – or for my soul?*

Although I didn't look at Bud's face, I knew he must be stricken by my strange and unprovoked attack. In one quick movement, he bolted from the room and rushed down the hallway to our bedroom. I heard him open the drawer to his nightstand, where I knew he kept a loaded pistol.

Dear God, I thought. *What have I done? Is he going to blow out his brains?* In an instant, the rage subsided. I hurried down the hallway and found him standing in the middle of our bedroom in his shorts, hanging up his dress pants. No gun was in sight.

"I'm sorry," I apologized quickly. "I didn't mean it the way it sounded." But I couldn't explain what I *did* mean and didn't want to try. I retreated to the living room. The hurt had been voiced. It could never be taken back. Words had been said in anger. One of the basic rules we always practiced in our marriage was, *Never speak in anger. Angry words cannot be retracted.*

But I didn't even know why I was so angry—or who I was angry at. I was consumed with anger and feelings of violence that I didn't understand.

As a child, I couldn't recall ever having a temper tantrum, but I had observed them in my younger sister when she was about three or four. Now I recalled the frustration on her young face as I watched her work through the tantrum while I held her down on the bed so she wouldn't hurt herself, until it passed. Was hers the same frustration I felt now? And was holding her down, against her will, the right thing to do? Now I doubted that it was. I didn't want to be held. I didn't even want to be touched.

It was a silent, wretched evening. We avoided each other's eyes and finally went to bed early. I didn't take the last estrogen tablet on the twenty-fifth day of my cycle and felt calmer the next morning.

Guarded in his comments, Bud declined breakfast. I knew he was walking a thin tightrope, trying to avoid conflict and confrontation, afraid he would set me off again.

"How are you feeling this morning?" he asked cautiously.

"I don't feel like exploding anymore, if that's what you're asking; I did *that* last night." I thought the problem needed to be confronted.

"Are you still bleeding?"

"I don't think so, or else it's very slight."

I had a brief nosebleed that morning but didn't mention it to him. I wondered if the combination of emotional outbursts, headaches, dizziness, driving over parking lot dividers (which I had done recently), and nosebleeds could be signs of a brain tumor.

Finally, when Bud got up to leave, I marshaled all my courage and asked, "Are you going to give me my good-bye hug this morning?" Would he even want to hug me again?

"You bet." He sounded cheerful for the first time as he set down his coffee cup on the counter and returned to embrace me in a smothering bear hug.

When he released me, I repeated once more, "I'm sorry." It was all I could manage. I kissed him good-bye.

That I had hurt him filled me with remorse. I was most sorry that I could not undo the hurt or even explain why I had said I blamed him. I went into the bathroom and began sorting clothes to wash.

I had sorted only a few items when he came back into the bathroom. He held out his arms and hugged me again. Then *he* began to cry— deep, heart-wrenching sobs. We just held each other for a moment. I ached with helplessness, knowing I had caused his grief but not knowing how to put things right again.

"I know it's hell for you too," I said finally, when he stopped crying. Without another word, he turned and left for work.

Accepting an idea rationally in my mind and accepting it emotionally in my heart are two very different concepts. Rationally, I knew I'd needed the surgery to live, but emotionally, had I really accepted it? I felt cheated—cheated out of the children we wanted and never had—and now never could have—and cheated out of the sexual gratification I might never experience again, but who remains duty-bound to continue having intercourse with a normal, sex-hungry male. Did I resent the fact that Bud was still intact while I was flawed—less than a woman? How could he know how I felt unless he too were neutered?

If I had been given more time to adjust to the idea of hysterectomy, would I have been more accepting of the surgery? I didn't know. Perhaps the depression wasn't mental. Perhaps it was hormonal.

I had a two o'clock appointment with Dr. Lance.

"How's everything going?" he greeted me cheerfully.

"Not very good," I replied. "I'm bleeding again, and I don't even want my husband to touch me." In an instant, I began sobbing, and I couldn't stop. I apologized for losing control.

His smile changed to an expression of grave concern as he listened sympathetically.

After examining me, Dr. Lance explained, "You still have a lot of granulation tissue. Granulation tissue is a form of scar tissue that bleeds easily and often takes a long time to heal. We can hasten the process with cryosurgery. It will freeze and destroy the scar tissue, thus preventing a recurrence of bleeding during intercourse. Internal healing is still taking place that could last for yet another month."

I complained about soreness around the upper edges of the incision, close to the navel.

"That is from the nerves and tissue still healing." Again, he cautioned, "Keep your stools soft and regular until healing is complete."

I ate bran flakes and fruit every day, but my bowel movements were erratic again. I blamed it on my irregular eating schedule while we were on vacation. Not only was constipation a constant annoyance, but I also felt bloated. My abdomen looked like a balloon, even though I'd gained only a pound and a half since my last visit. I decided to return to the stool softener/laxative and try some tummy-tightening exercises.

We discussed my melancholia.

"There is no pleasure in sex for me anymore," I wailed. "Will I ever get back to normal? I don't even want my husband to touch me."

"As long as you're still having pain, you aren't going to have much pleasure," he sympathized. "And you have very definite symptoms of depression. Depression will also lower your sex drive." The pleasant feelings, he reassured me, would probably return when all these other problems were resolved.

Much later I realized the full importance of his analysis of my condition: *you do not feel loving when you are depressed or in pain.*

We discussed my hormone regulation. My breasts weren't sore, nor did I have symptoms of estrogen overdose, so he didn't recommend changing the estrogen dosage or frequency. I had mentioned that a friend said her doctor put her on an every-other-day estrogen regimen. Instead, he advised adding 10 milligrams of progesterone for the last ten days of each twenty-five-day cycle (days sixteen to twenty-five) to balance out the mood swings. He wrote a prescription.

"If that doesn't help," he counseled, "I'll have to recommend psychiatric help for you." Although I didn't relish the thought of visiting a "shrink," I had reached a point where I was willing to try anything.

"I got the subpoena for your file from the Arizona Board of Medical Examiners," he said, almost as an afterthought. "In fact, they have your file right now. I can't even refer to it."

"I'm sorry I didn't have a chance to forewarn you," I apologized. "I wrote the letter just before we left on vacation. Their reply came while we were gone. I wrote both you and Dr. Fields as soon as I read their letter. You'll probably get it today or tomorrow. Quite frankly, I didn't expect them to act so fast."

As I was leaving his office, my file from the medical board was returned.

I felt happy knowing the medical examiner's office was working on the investigation. It gave me hope that perhaps my surgery was not entirely in vain. Perhaps the misdeeds of Arcadia Clinic would be exposed, and they would be put out of business. Hopefully, my phone call to Betty had not given her the alert she needed to destroy incriminating evidence in my file. But perhaps she was so ignorant about what might be incriminating that she wouldn't even know what evidence to destroy. I hoped she had been lulled into thinking I would not pursue action against them. Almost a year had passed since I last visited their clinic.

Later in the day, when I called our neighbor Mary to let her know we were back from vacation, she asked, "Did you notice we've taken down the "For Sale" sign? We decided to stay in the neighborhood for another four years, until all the kids have graduated from high school."

"That's the best news I've heard in a long time," I replied. That, coupled with the news that Arcadia Clinic was being investigated, brightened my day. I felt my life starting to turn around and change for the better.

Bud came home from work as I stood at the sink, preparing dinner.

"We need to talk about last night," he said. I was glad he'd broached the subject. It needed to be confronted before it had a chance to fester. We needed to share our feelings and understand each other's thoughts.

"You scared me last night," he began.

"I scared myself," I replied. "I was totally out of control. I didn't know what I was capable of doing and was afraid of what I might do."

"I went into the bedroom and unloaded all the handguns and hid them—and the bullets," he confessed.

I laughed. "And I thought I had hurt you so deeply that you'd gone back there to blow out your brains. When I heard you rummaging around in the nightstand for your gun, I was scared for you. I think that is what brought me out of the rage."

"Next time it happens, God forbid, what can I do to help you?" he asked. "I knew you were sinking into depression. I could see it at supper."

"I was so afraid you'd say something to me in the restaurant and that I'd lose control and go stark raving mad right there."

"I just wanted to get you home to talk to you," he said. "That's why I was so irritated when the waitress took so long to bring the bill."

I hadn't even noticed the long wait or that he was irritated. I thought he acted very calm.

"I wanted to let you know how I felt," I explained. "That's why I told you I thought I was sinking into a depression that I might not get out of. Do you remember what you said? You said, 'No, you aren't.' That's when I went berserk. I thought, *Do I have to become a stark raving maniac before you'll admit I still have a problem?* Dr. Lance had to say cancer and surgery before you'd admit I had a problem that needed surgery. We both thought surgery would solve the problem once and for all. Well, it hasn't! *I still have a problem!* We need to face that fact. We need to admit it. We need to confront it."

"What I meant," Bud said defensively, "was that I wouldn't let you sink into that kind of depression, that we'd get you the help you needed *before* you reached that stage, even if we have to spend every cent we've ever saved."

(Later, I thought that was one of the most loving things Bud had ever said to me. My close-with-the-dollar husband was willing to spend every dime we had to help me get well.)

"I guess, in a way, I blamed you for talking me into having the surgery before you had all the facts," I said. "You wouldn't even read the book I gave you about the complications and side effects. And now, the surgery may not have ended my problem; it may be just the beginning of another problem." I had regained my composure. Tonight, I was not crying.

"I *did* read the book," he insisted, "but later. You probably didn't see me. I still say that if the surgery was needed to save your life; it was necessary. I would do it again."

"Actually, once I gave it more thought, I realized *you* didn't talk me into having the surgery. Remember? That was the one decision I said

I had to make for myself. And when I finally made it, I was at peace with it. I guess God knew it was necessary that we both knew I had to make that decision—so I couldn't blame you."

"What should I do if you get into that kind of mood again?" he asked, still bewildered. "I don't know how to react."

"I don't know either," I confessed. "I don't understand what is happening to me, and I can't seem to cope with it. It scared me because I knew what I was doing; I just couldn't *stop*. I felt possessed. I guess the best thing to do is what you did. Don't rock the boat. Give me a wide berth and hope I can work my way out of it. If I knew what was causing the problem, the solution would be easier to find. What I felt was *rage*—that's the closest I can come to a diagnosis. I guess I need to learn what the rage is directed at. It's probably still directed at Arcadia Clinic and all the doctors who let my condition deteriorate for so long, necessitating such extensive surgery."

I had trusted the practitioners at Arcadia Clinic, placing my faith in Dr. Jim and Betty and their medical knowledge. I had been led to believe that Betty was qualified to treat my medical problems—and I *had* believed it. The rage was directed not only at her but at my own culpability—my own stupidity. I considered myself to be an intelligent, knowledgeable person, but I had been duped. I had been betrayed. Like Judas, Betty had planted the kiss of death and left me to carry the cross.

Talking to Bud now, I said, "I only know that when you left the room, it broke the spell. My attention was distracted from myself to you. I guess it was the right thing to do."

Brain tumor still lurked in the recesses of my mind—the mood swings, the splitting headaches. Recently I'd unknowingly driven over a parking lot divider, getting my car hung up on it. I had needed help getting the wheels off the cement block. Were the previous episodes of clouded vision and mental dullness other signs of brain tumor?

"Perhaps you read too much," Mary suggested one day as we were having coffee. I knew what she was trying to tell me: if I hadn't read so many hematology books, I wouldn't have known my symptoms could indicate a brain tumor, and perhaps, I wouldn't have gotten myself worked up over that possibility. But I had read. And I did know. If I could ever become well again, I had to dispel all my fears. I needed to find the real cause for my symptoms, even if it was a brain tumor.

What else could cause these personality changes so unlike the "real" me? I was the original Pollyanna—or so some of my post-college roommates called me. They might not have meant it as a compliment, but I was flattered by that description, feeling that I always looked on the bright side of life, even when there was no bright side. Adversity had never worried me—before.

Knowledge was not something to fear; it was something to benefit humankind. How could my research be detrimental?

That night, I went to bed early. I still tired easily. The next morning I awoke with a splitting headache. Bud reminded me that it was the third day after flying when the inner ear problems had started. I began taking antihistamines, hoping to ward off a recurrence of the dreadful dizzy spells.

CHAPTER 21

CRYOSURGERY

On Dr. Lance's advice, I took a stool softener/laxative before retiring, and contrary to my previous experience, the next day I couldn't stay out of the bathroom, almost bordering on diarrhea. I thought my intestines must have been blocked—clear up to my esophagus.

Terrible headaches still plagued me, with pressure building at the base of my skull where the head joins the spinal column; repeating symptoms of my vacation illness. As a precaution, I again took the anti-vertigo medicine.

By mid-afternoon, though sickeningly nauseated, I had no dizziness. Finally, I called Dr. Field's office, explaining my previous bout with what I thought to be an inner ear infection and my fear that it was returning.

Dr. Fields was out of the office, but one of the other doctors on staff, believing I had a bacterial rather than a viral infection, prescribed a strong antibiotic. By the time Bud came home from work with the prescription, I had entered the vomiting stage. After taking the medicine, I returned to bed. The nausea persisted, but if I lay very still, I could control the vomiting. The vertigo never materialized.

I continued to take the antibiotic as prescribed, but by noon the next day, still feeling poorly, I called Dr. Fields's office again, asking if I should also take the anti-vertigo medicine as a preventive measure.

Neither he nor I was completely convinced I had an inner ear infection. He advised me to come to the office.

"How are you feeling?" he asked, entering the examination room.

"Lousy," I replied, handing him a typed list of all my symptoms, along with the dates from the time I first experienced the spells of dizziness, vomiting, and nausea. He examined me but could find nothing amiss. He suspected the flu and told me to discontinue the antibiotic, which he thought might be irritating my stomach, a frequent side effect of this drug.

"How do I know my thyroid dosage is correct?" I queried now. "Arcadia Clinic misdiagnosed and mistreated everything else. How do I know they didn't overdose me on thyroid too?"

"I can order a thyroid profile," he offered.

Grasping at straws now, I said, "When I was in Wisconsin on vacation, I learned one of my first cousins has lupus. Do you think I need a third lupus test? Maybe mine has been in remission, and now it's out. From what I've read, lupus in remission may not give a positive reading."

"That's true," he said, "but I don't think you have lupus."

"Also," I continued, hoping to provide Dr. Fields with additional, helpful information, "my dad just had hip replacement surgery for osteoarthritis."

"You may have an arthritic condition," he conceded. "We'll run another sedimentation rate with the CBC."

I told him my bones still ached, but it might be from the bone scraping during surgery.

Two days later, I felt decidedly better; only some lightheadedness and headache still remained. Dr. Fields's nurse called to report my hemoglobin test was normal: 13.8.

"I guess I can stop taking the iron now," I said. She agreed.

The sedimentation rate, however, was up to thirty-two. I wondered if the flu could have caused that increase, or if I had another problem. The T4 thyroid profile was 6.0—normal.

"Do not change your medication," the nurse instructed, referring to the Thyrolar. As I looked back through my medical files, I found the T4 test Betty had ordered the year before. It also was 6.0—before she decided to increase the Thyrolar dosage from one grain to two grains per day. I needed to question Dr. Fields about that the next time I saw him.

On Sunday I read an article in the local newspaper about PMS (premenstrual syndrome), which is caused by hormonal imbalance. It listed many of my symptoms: abdominal bloating, backache, weight gain, breast tenderness, acne, constipation, cravings for sweet and salty foods (a new symptom I'd noticed since surgery, mostly toward the end of my cycle), headache, irritability, fatigue, lethargy, tension, anxiety, depression, and violence. One of the treatments for PMS was the administration of progesterone.

When I visited Dr. Lance for the cryosurgery, I greeted him with, "You are one super doctor."

"What brought on that compliment?" he asked, flattered.

I showed him the article on PMS that I'd cut from Sunday's paper. He scanned it rapidly. "You may also need B6 supplements," he said thoughtfully. "Get the 50-milligram tablets. Take one with breakfast and one with supper. You may need to increase the dosage to two tablets twice a day, but don't take more than 200 milligrams a day."

Later, as I researched vitamin B6, I learned it was found in quantity only in foods most people seldom eat: liver, brewer's yeast, and wheat germ. A negligible amount is found in egg yolks and a small amount in bananas and yogurt. A high-protein diet, such as I had been advised to follow for hypoglycemia, can destroy B6 in the system. Lack of vitamin B6 can be a factor in causing inner ear infections. Now I was really impressed with my doctor.

The cryosurgery proved to be nothing to dread. When I was escorted into the examining room, a metal tank, similar to a large oxygen tank, was already in the room. This contained the gas used for the freezing process.

Before surgery, with the use of a speculum to open the vagina and a magnifying mirror, Dr. Lance showed me the granulation tissue, located at the very end of the vagina, where the cervix had been removed. Right in the middle of the healed incision was what looked like a very large, red, blood-filled pimple.

"Granulation tissue," Dr. Lance said, "is quite sensitive to irritation and would probably continue to bleed with intercourse, if left untreated. Eventually, it will heal completely and disappear, but sometimes that takes many months. The freezing process simply hastens the healing. New tissue will form that is not granulation tissue."

The procedure was not uncomfortable. I imagined him to be "airbrushing" the tissue with the gas he used during the cryosurgery. First, he would airbrush, then allow it to warm, and then he would airbrush again. All I felt was a small amount of internal cramping, as he warned I would. The process was repeated several times until he felt all the granulation tissue had been destroyed. He said I might feel pain or weakness afterward, but I did not.

"There will be a discharge for a few days," he warned, "and it might be quite foul-smelling. I'll recheck you in a week to see if we need to do any touch-up cryosurgery."

"I'm starting to feel peppier and more normal again," I commented, "My hemoglobin is up to 13.8, but my sedimentation rate is also high—thirty-two."

"The sed rate is one of the least accurate medical tests," he said—a fact I already knew from my hematology research. But why did all my sed test results continue to be above normal?

Since I now felt better, I decided to stop worrying about the possibility of lupus.

When we arrived home from vacation, the book Laura promised to send, *Life without Limits: The Message of Mark's Gospel* by Lloyd J. Ogilvie, waited with the mail.

Each morning, I read a chapter from the book, along with the accompanying companion chapter from the book of Mark in the Bible, an in-depth study of Mark's Gospel. I found it so interesting and rewarding that I wanted to ration myself to a single chapter each day, so I could absorb the message slowly and completely. Was God telling me I needed to put aside some quiet time each day for Him? I also felt a need to probe the whole Bible in more depth, to saturate my soul with scripture. Perhaps that was for a future need.

The Gospel lesson from Mark 2—the story about the man who had been let down through the ceiling to be healed—especially touched me, particularly when Jesus asks, "Which is easier to say: 'Your sins are forgiven,' or to say, 'Rise, take up your bed and walk'?"

It finally made sense to me now; I knew the answer to that question. While many people, including doctors, are credited with curing illness, God alone can cure (forgive) sin. It was a life-changing revelation.

CHAPTER 22

"SOMETHING IS *STILL* WRONG"

On Friday, October 15, 1982, I visited Dr. Fields again. It had been almost a year since my first visit to his office.

"My blood count is down again, isn't it?" I greeted him as he entered the examining room. It wasn't really a fair question. His nurse had already told me it was lower than the previous high of 13.8.

"It's 12.3," he replied.

During the past several weeks, I'd felt a drop in my energy levels, so I strongly suspected a dropping blood count might be the reason. Although not completely surprised by the news, I was devastated to learn I was still battling anemia. The surgery had not solved the problem.

"The seizures have returned too," I reported.

"Seizures? What do you mean seizures?" he questioned, looking at me with his intense gaze. His eyes burned into my body like two pieces of glowing black coal. I only wished they possessed x-ray vision and could look into my body to discover the source of the problem.

"I don't really know how to describe them," I replied. Resignation crept into my voice. "I feel foggy, mentally dull, spaced out, out of focus. Sometimes I feel like I'm becoming senile. It's the only word I can think of to adequately describe the condition—memory lapses, forgetfulness, and impaired concentration. They don't always last very long, usually not more than a half hour. I can't see any pattern to them. Sometimes, they come in the morning, sometimes in the afternoon, and sometimes after supper."

"Anything else?" he probed.

"My eyes feel like they aren't focusing properly, yet I can see to read. But I don't always comprehend what I'm reading. I feel like I'm looking through the split in my bifocals. They're the same symptoms I had when I first visited you last October. And I still have some slight headaches, dizziness, and mild nausea, especially when I turn my head rapidly."

"What do you mean?"

"When I turn my head suddenly or look up really fast, I get dizzy. Sometimes, I feel like I'm going to fall over backward unless I hold on to something. Once in a while, I get momentarily sick to my stomach, but it usually doesn't last long."

"Have you ever had a brain scan?"

"No."

"If the mental dullness doesn't clear, perhaps you should consider having one." He made it sound like a routine diagnostic procedure, not something urgent, but he hadn't made the gynecological exam sound urgent either. Did he, too, suspect a brain tumor but didn't want to alarm me?

"Is there *any* possibility that I could have lupus?" I asked. More than anything, I wanted to find a cause for the anemia—any cause short of cancer.

While I lacked medical knowledge, I knew my symptoms better than anyone else. By sharing my theories about the illnesses that fit my symptoms, I reasoned Dr. Fields could point out the medical errors in my conclusions. And now, he did just that.

"Your last ANA test was normal," he reassured me, "and you don't have enough other symptoms to indicate lupus."

I accepted his evaluation—a giant step forward for me to trust my doctor's judgment. "Could it be hormonal imbalance?" I probed. "I'm still having some depression. It seems more pronounced toward the end of my cycle—about day twenty-three on estrogen. But last time, day twenty-four seemed less severe. I can't see a pattern to it."

"How much estrogen are you taking?"

"0.625 milligrams."

"That's awfully strong," he commented. Then, as if catching himself, he asked, "Did they remove either of your ovaries with the hysterectomy?"

"They took *everything*," I replied dully, thinking back to the surgery report. Dr. Lance had said, "With the endometriosis being so extensive, there was really nothing worth saving."

Later, I reflected that if Dr. Fields thought the 0.625 milligram dose was strong, what would he have thought about the 2.5 milligram dosage of estrogen that Betty prescribed before the surgery when I still had both ovaries?

"How much progesterone do you take?" he asked.

"Ten milligrams the last ten days of each cycle."

"That's a normal dosage."

"I'm still having breast tenderness," I confessed. "When I first started the progesterone, I thought I was a young woman again. My breasts ballooned out like a teenager's. But lately they haven't felt so full."

"You could try a half dosage of estrogen for a month," he suggested. "Try to see if that improves your condition. Your tablets are scored. Just break them in half. If need be, we can also try half doses of progesterone later."

I told him leg pains continued to plague me.

"These might be from an osteoarthritis condition," he suggested, and the constipation, still bothersome, could be caused by an irritable colon. "Use stool softeners, and keep yourself regular."

"I do use stool softeners," I said, "and I eat bran flakes every day." Frustrated and at my wit's end, nothing seemed to help.

"Which stool softener are you using?"

I mentioned the brand Dr. Lance had recommended.

"Why are you using such a harsh one?" he asked.

"Dr. Lance recommended it after surgery," I explained. "He said I had to keep my stools soft."

Dr. Fields suggested the names of several stool softeners that did not contain laxatives.

"What was my last thyroid reading?" I asked.

"Your T4 was 6.4. That's in the normal range."

"But my T4 was 6.0 before Betty increased my Thyrolar dosage from one grain to two grains a day," I said. Suspicious now, I asked, "Is 6.0 also in a normal range?"

He agreed it was but suggested, "We can reduce your dosage to one grain daily and do another T4 reading in three months."

When I started taking Thyrolar, Betty had ordered a small dose (a quarter of a grain). As years passed, she gradually increased the dosage until I took two grains daily—eight times stronger. Only recently I learned the device she had used to check my thyroid function—a photomotogram—was an outdated instrument not considered reliable since the 1930s.

I wondered if I'd ever needed thyroid medication or if this was just one more of Betty's shots in the dark to pep me up and address my complaints of fatigue. Had she revved up my metabolism so that now I had hyperthyroidism (too much thyroid hormone)? Only I knew which methods had been used to diagnose my condition, which medications were put into my body and in what quantities—all at her direction.

The more I thought about it, the more I reasoned that none of it was good. Did holistic medicine first create illness and then claim to treat it? And why would she double the dosage when my thyroid test was normal? Wasn't I getting sick fast enough to satisfy her? Had I become her private little lab rat?

Dr. Fields checked my heart, lungs, lymph glands, and spleen. Everything seemed to be normal. He made no effort to conceal the fact that he was plainly puzzled by my case, although for my sake he tried to be optimistic.

"Do you have any idea what is causing my anemia?" I finally asked

"Anemia may be normal for you," he replied, repeating a previous statement.

"Something is still wrong!" I wanted to scream. *"Something is wrong with my body, and now, something is wrong with my brain!"* How could I get him to understand? But I didn't scream. I didn't even voice those fears. I remained calm and said nothing. That, in itself, was progress.

"We'll check you again in three months, unless you have more problems." It was his polite way of ending the appointment. But what more was there to say? To the best of his ability, he had answered all my questions and tried to calm my fears. I still did not know what was causing the anemia, but I was certain of one thing: it wasn't *normal* for me.

During the week of October 18, our church women's convention was scheduled at Asilomar campgrounds in California. I was registered to attend. Dr. Fields had given his consent for me to go, even though the trip involved a fatiguing sixteen-hour bus ride. In order to conserve my energy, I brought along sleeping pills and slept at least four hours on the moving bus, both coming and going. In previous years, I had not slept at all.

Still, the convention caused me to be fraught with fatigue—a sign that I was not totally recovered, even though six months had passed since my surgery. As a member of the convention's office staff, much of my behind-the-scenes work of typing and printing materials for the next day's sessions was performed in the late evening or early morning hours. Still, I managed to squeeze in six hours of sleep each night. Insomnia no longer plagued me. Almost as soon as my head touched the pillow, I fell asleep. Normally, six hours of sound sleep would have sufficed, but now, it never was enough.

One night I walked into the convention office about ten o'clock, after the evening's closing session. I knew I was tired when the thin carpeting on the office floor looked inviting. I lay down on the carpet, behind the registration desk, hoping I wasn't too visible. I was almost asleep a half hour later when the women arrived with the materials I needed to type for the next day's session.

I slept on the bus during the long ride back home, but arrived exhausted. However, during the convention, I'd made a decision. For my own peace of mind, I had to have that brain scan.

CHAPTER 23

QUICKSAND

On Monday, November 8, after feeling exceptionally well for the past week, I began to think my mental fuzziness had been caused by the thyroid overdose, and now, after taking an adjusted lower dose for more than three weeks, I didn't need the CT scan after all. But this morning when I awoke and turned over in bed, the room went into an all-too-familiar rapid spin. Remembering past dizzy spells, I lay very still. True to form, the spinning slowed and stopped, but left me nauseated.

The urge to empty my bowels coaxed me out of bed. Once emptied, feeling somewhat better, I rejoined Bud in bed. Ten or fifteen minutes later, I repeated the process. After a while, I felt better so I got up, brushed my teeth, and started to dress, only to have another sudden wave of nausea wash over me, forcing me back to bed, fully clothed.

I asked Bud to call Dr. Fields from work. "Ask him if he still wants me to have the brain scan." My head felt ready to explode from pressure. I wondered if it would be advisable to inject dye into it, especially if fluid buildup caused the pain. It was day twenty-five of my cycle.

Lying very still on my back, I waited for the nausea to pass. A short time later, I slowly turned over onto my left side and fell asleep. I slept like I had been drugged and woke at nine thirty to the telephone ringing.

It was Bud. "You have an appointment with Dr. Fields at ten o'clock," he said. "Mary will drive you there. Dr. Fields wants you to have the brain scan, but he wants to see you first." Bud had been busy making arrangements.

By the time Mary arrived, the dizziness had passed. Except for feeling weak and hungry from no breakfast, I now felt fine.

Dr. Fields checked my heart, lungs, ears, and eyes (for internal pressure) but found nothing out of the ordinary.

"I've been feeling great this past week," I reported. "Yesterday I even helped dig out a mulberry tree root." Our mulberry trees had died. We needed to remove them. "We didn't push it. We worked a while and rested a while. I didn't feel like I had overexerted, yet I've noticed these 'seizures' often occur after physical exertion."

He ran his prickly wheel over various parts of my body, checking nerve responses. The sensations in my right and left forearms seemed different. "The right side seems less sensitive," I commented.

"Everything appears fine," he said after completing his examination, "but I want a neurologist to see you after the brain scan, whether the scan is normal or not."

To me, these dizzy spells now seemed like an omen of hope. Just before leaving, I commented, "I think the end is getting very near."

"Oh, I don't believe that," Dr. Fields replied quickly.

As I left his office, I suddenly realized how he must have interpreted my comment, so explained to his nurse. "Please tell Dr. Fields what I meant is that I think the *search* is coming to an end—not the end of *me*."

My attitude had changed from a person who wanted no surgery performed on her body to one who looked forward to brain surgery, if that would relieve the symptoms now threatening both my body and my mind.

The brain scan was a simple procedure. Bud came with me to the nuclear medicine section of Mercy Hospital. I felt like I had become a regular customer there.

The procedure didn't require changing into a hospital gown. I climbed onto a moveable table that looked like a piece of it was missing. The attendant strapped my head onto a padded holder; a wedge cushion was inserted under my knees to keep them in a bent position. A blanket covered me. Was it to protect me from the radiation or the cold? The cold, I decided; the x-ray room was chilly.

The machine looked like an old-fashioned outdoor oven, except the surface was gleaming metal instead of stone. The table moved slowly forward. I went head first into the opening, seemingly on a conveyor belt, until the scanning device was at the base of my brain. Myriad tiny lights in a semicircle pattern scanned the skull. When completed, the table moved again, drawing me a short distance out of the machine. The procedure was repeated, scanning the next portion of my brain, until the entire brain area was scanned. The top of my head was scanned last.

When I asked the technician, she said the x-ray did not scan the neck vertebrae. Most of my pressure seemed to be located at the very base of my skull, where my head joined the spinal column at the neck vertebrae.

Following the initial set of x-rays, radioactive iodine dripped into a vein in my arm. It was not as fast as the IV pyelogram drip, so I didn't experience the warm flush I had with the kidney test. Again the scanning procedure started at the base of my brain and worked upward. Both brain scans, with and without dye, took about ten minutes.

Several friends had told me they'd discovered they were claustrophobic while taking this test, but it didn't bother me. I closed my eyes. If it had lasted longer, I could have slept; the lulling buzz of the scanning mechanism was relaxing. "Don't move your head," the technician instructed. How could I? It was strapped down.

Toward the end of the test, I felt slightly chilled. Whether from the cold room, the radioactive dye, or the emphasis on remaining motionless, I didn't know. Afterward, my teeth hurt. *Do metal fillings attract radioactivity?* I wondered. I would have had no problem driving myself home, but Bud drove.

By nightfall, the dizziness had mostly passed, although I still felt tired, so I went to bed early. At one thirty, the need to empty my bladder woke me. Since the radioactive iodine is excreted through the kidneys,

I decided not to ignore this call and was dismayed to find the dizziness had returned. It seemed worse when I lay on my right side or when I lay flat on my back. So I carefully turned over to my left side.

The next morning as I got up carefully, Bud said, "MS." I looked at him quizzically. He explained, "MS—move slow." But *multiple sclerosis* had popped into my mind. Was God preparing me for yet another phase of this illness? Once upright, the dizziness and nausea diminished, but the fullness and pressure in the back of my head remained.

After lunch on Wednesday, I called Dr. Fields's office. They hadn't called me, and I anxiously awaited the test results. "Your report is normal," the nurse said.

On to the next step. She gave me the name of a neurologist they recommended. I made an appointment for November 18, a week away.

After getting myself hyped up for brain surgery, the "normal" report hit me with a staggering blow. While my family and friends took the attitude, "Praise the Lord," depression dogged me. How much longer would the "not knowing" continue? I resented having my body subjected to so much radiation with no answers yet. How many more tests lay ahead? I feared the necessity of a spinal tap to check for fluid in the brain, and questioned whether I also needed a CAT scan of my entire body to check for bone cancer.

> **Wednesday, November 10, 1983**
> I am still filled with *rage* toward my quack doctors, who I blame for my affliction, not only because they didn't properly treat my condition but also because they indiscriminately overdosed me with unneeded medicines and vitamins, possibly creating the physical and mental conditions I now suffer. I had hoped a brain tumor would give me the solid evidence I needed to put this medical group out of business, but now a brain tumor had been eliminated.

I called Dr. Lance, asking if hormonal imbalance could be causing the dizziness and nausea. He said it could cause nausea, but he didn't know about the dizziness. He suggested I increase the B6 dosage to 100 milligrams in the morning and 100 milligrams with supper but no more than 200 milligrams a day. I confessed I had only been taking one 50-milligram tablet a day, often forgetting the second one at suppertime. "Dr. Fields recommended I reduce the estrogen by half because of my breast tenderness," I said.

He disagreed, suggesting I return to the 0.625-milligram level. "If you continue to experience breast tenderness, you might want to reduce the progesterone to 0.5 milligrams a day for the last ten days of your cycle," he added.

Currently, I felt better during my five days off. My body seemed to need this time off from hormones each month. Was I still getting too much?

Thursday, November 11, 1982
Last night I went to bed at nine o'clock, falling fast asleep before ten. To sleep so deeply and so quickly after retiring is unusual for me. I didn't even hear Bud come to bed. Today, after a good night's sleep, I am in a better frame of mind.

We called my brother, Harold, and his family last night to report the brain scan results. After talking with them, it dawned on me that even if a brain tumor had been found, it probably wasn't the cause of the anemia, just as the hysterectomy hadn't solve that problem. The less surgery required, the better, I decided. Who really wants to have brain surgery? My spirits began to lift.

I recalled a dream I'd had the last night at convention. I was walking on the edge of a swamp when suddenly I stepped off into quicksand. As I began to sink and flounder, I remembered that a person should not struggle against quicksand. Struggling only causes you to sink deeper faster. So I tried to remain calm, knowing that Bud was nearby, and he would pull me out. I glanced toward where he stood on solid ground. He reached out to grab me, catching my forearms, trying to pull me from the muck. But by this time, my hands and arms were covered with the slimy goo; his hands slipped off. He tried again and again, but my arms kept sliding out of his grasp. He couldn't get a firm hold or enough leverage to pull me free. My body was sinking deeper and deeper. I was being swallowed by this muddy hole. And as much as he wanted to, Bud couldn't help me; he couldn't pull me free.

I woke up. It was only four o'clock, but I couldn't get back to sleep. The dream had troubled my mind.

Remembering the dream, now I wondered, *Am I being swallowed, sucked up into some kind of evil over which neither Bud nor I have any control? And if so, what is it?*

CHAPTER 24

TEST THE SPIRITS

Tuesday, November 16, 1982

The seizures, or spells, are becoming more frequent and more severe. Although I have a semblance of clear-headedness for several hours after waking, the dizziness and nausea permeates most of my day. My mind feels like it is in a constant conflict or battle to keep the symptoms under control, as one does when fighting to control the urge to vomit, and I feel that I am losing this battle.

By mid-afternoon, the pressure at the base of my skull builds to explosive proportions. If I lie completely still for an hour, sometimes part of the pressure is relieved, seemingly caused by tension in the neck muscles. Lying down relaxes those muscles.

Today is day three of my cycle. My sleep pattern has changed in recent months. Normally, I'm a light insomniac sleeper; now I fall into a deep, almost drugged-like state. Nothing wakes me—not even Bud coming to bed late or his getting up in the middle of the night to let the cat out. Only when my internal alarm clock goes off at six o'clock do I wake. Then I am wide awake.

In *Your Thyroid Gland, Fact and Fiction*,[12] Joel I. Hamburger, MD, states that the thyroid pill you take today does not make you feel better

---

[12] Joel I. Hamburger, MD. *Your Thyroid Gland—Fact and Fiction* (Springfield, IL: Thomas, 1970).

tomorrow; it makes you feel better three weeks from today. I wonder if the thyroid pill I'm *not* taking has finally allowed my body to slow down enough to rest. Insomnia may be the symptom of an overactive thyroid.

Yesterday, the dizziness was worse when I looked up or had to reach above my head, as when I stretched to get a box of noodles off the top cupboard shelf.

I succumb to lying down more frequently, but the pressure does not cease; my neck muscles are unable to relax. I wonder if the parathyroid gland at the base of the brain may somehow be involved. By nine o'clock this morning, I quit the mind-over-matter struggle to control the dizziness and nausea and went to bed. Lying flat on my back still aggravates the vertigo. If I move slowly to the left, the nausea subsides; then I can shift to the right side—the side I usually sleep on. When these spells occur, the right side is more sensitive to motion, whereas lying on the left side helps quell the motion sickness.

I hope the symptoms are becoming clear-cut and repetitious enough that the neurologist can make an instant diagnosis and put me back on the road to good health. Since reducing the thyroid medication by one grain a day, my left leg has pained less, but enough twinges remain to remind me there is still a problem, now accompanied by a dull, throbbing pain in my left hip joint.

In the past, I always considered myself a spiritual person yet found it easy to ignore good spiritual habits. Reading the Bible and praying for others on a regular basis were activities I often put off. But now I find myself drawn to the Bible. I want to immerse myself in its comforting words, chapter after chapter. I can't seem to get enough of God's Word and am especially drawn to First, Second, and Third John, which counsels, "I write to you, not because you do not know the truth, but because you know it, and know that no lie is of the truth" (1 John 2:21 RSV).

My holistic healers had lied to me. They were not holy healers; they did not speak the truth. They did not heal in the name of God. Also, I read, "Who are the children of the devil: whoever does not do right is not of God" (1 John 3:10b RSV), and "Do not believe every spirit, but test the spirits to see whether they are from God, for many false prophets have gone out into the world" (1 John 4:1 RSV).

I found myself reading and rereading these three books from the Bible over and over again. "He, who does not love, does not know God; for God is love" (1 John 4:8 RSV), and "There is no fear in love, but perfect love casts out fear" (1 John 4:18a RSV). Was my real battle with the devil and the forces of evil in the world? Had holistic medicine taken control of my spirit with its subtle sinister seduction?

As I realized my own need for prayer, I also felt the need to pray for others. *A better, more prayerful world begins with me*, I decided.

Friday, November 19, 1982
Yesterday I saw Dr. Johnson, the neurologist. He took my history and performed some tests for reflex action. "Your reflexes appear to be normal," he said. I recalled the number of photomotograms Betty had used to test my reflexes. Dr. Johnson didn't perform a single one. Was the photomotogram just another holistic device they used to create a feeling of well-being, to make me believe they were helping my body?

When Bud and I arrived in Dr. Johnson's office, I looked on the magazine table for something to read while we waited and noticed a postcard invitation to a Parkinson's disease party at Arcadia Clinic. *Should I be consulting this neurologist if he associates with members of Arcadia Clinic?* I wondered. And did Dr. Fields send me here because he suspected I might have Parkinson's disease? I dismissed the thought, wondering if Arcadia Clinic experimented with Parkinson's disease too. First they caused the condition; then they pretended to treat it. Would they stoop so low?

The day before the EEG test, I was told, "Eat regular meals but no stimulants—no coffee, tea, cola, etc. Wash your head twenty-four hours before taking the test." On the day of the test, I experienced a slight fullness in the back of my head but no spinning or nausea. I wondered if the test would be conclusive if all my symptoms were absent.

I've been on 0.625 milligrams of estrogen and 200 milligrams of B6 for the past five days and still question whether my problem is hormonal.

Dr. Johnson asked about my mental state. It seems every doctor considers depression as a cause for my symptoms. Even I am beginning to question whether or not it is. I am getting tired of visiting doctor after doctor, learning nothing new—that, in itself, is enough to make a person depressed.

"Are you under any stress?" Dr. Johnson asked.

"No."

He chuckled. "I'd like to get your secret."

"I finally decided there is nothing I can do," I explained. "It's now up to my doctors and God."

"At least I'm in good company," he joked. "The normal CT scan ruled out brain tumor, brain hemorrhage, and hydrocephalus—an accumulation of water on the brain." I was glad to hear the last pronouncement. It meant I wouldn't need a spinal tap. Yet all the normal results were becoming depressants in themselves because they indicated the search must continue.

I'd reached a point of resignation again—not acceptance but resignation—just as I had before surgery. I wished we could find *something*—anything, even cancer, something to fight. Something to identify; something we could put a name to. Occasionally, I wondered if depression *was* the real problem. Then I'd ask myself, *If it is, why am I so lucid in my reasoning?*

We discussed hypoglycemia.

"I've had controlled hypoglycemia for sixteen years," I said. "In my estimation, the spells don't indicate hypoglycemia. I have not changed my diet. I avoid sugar."

"Do you have cancer of any kind?"

"Not that anyone can find." It unnerved me that my doctors kept asking *me* if I had cancer. That's what *they* were supposed to be diagnosing. If I knew I had cancer, we'd have something to treat.

Dr. Johnson and I discussed injuries to my brain.

When I was young, I had been in two automobile accidents that caused severe blows to my head. At age seven, a goose-egg bump had been raised on the back of my head, right side. I pointed to the spot. At age fourteen, I had hit the car windshield so forcefully with my forehead that it bent my metal-framed glasses.

"Did you black out?"

"No, I don't think I was ever out completely, only stunned for a minute."

"Have you ever had seizures or blackouts?"

"If you are wondering about psychomotor seizures, I don't think I have them. My sister-in-law has them. We have compared notes. My symptoms are not the same as hers."

"How's that?"

"She blacks out completely for small periods of time and loses some portion of conversations. I never black out. I can hear the person speaking but sometimes can't assimilate the information rapidly or with understanding. I can hear what is being said; I just can't absorb its meaning. Mine is like a time-delayed reaction. If I have a chance to digest the information and turn it over in my mind for a while, then I can process it. It's the *instant processing* that seems to be the problem."

"Maybe your sister-in-law's seizures last for several seconds, even minutes, while yours are shorter, lasting only a second or two," he theorized.

It sounded logical at the time, but later I questioned why some of the mental fuzziness or cloudiness lasted for longer periods—up to a half hour or more. Was I experiencing a multitude of mini-seizures one after the other, each one of short duration?

"I'd like you to have an EEG [electroencephalogram]," he said finally.

"Okay." I nodded in agreement. I had expected that to be the next step. It was scheduled for ten thirty the next morning.

According to my instructions, I was supposed to fall asleep during part of the test and had been advised to stay up late the night before. I read until eleven o'clock, well past my normal nine o'clock bedtime, and awoke at five thirty. Before my appointment, I vacuumed the floors, washed last night's supper dishes, and completed other housework, hoping to fatigue myself so I'd sleep during the test. But now I felt more wide awake than ever.

"There's no way you're going to get me to fall asleep during the day," I warned the technician who administered the test. "I'm just not a day sleeper and haven't been since I was four years old, unless I was sick."

The EEG was painless. I lay on a hard bed with a comfortable pillow. The nurse swabbed the spots on my head with alcohol before attaching twenty-one electrodes.

"I didn't know a person had nerves in the ear lobes," I commented as she attached one there.

"That measures your pulse rate," she explained.

When all the electrodes were placed, I was instructed to get into a comfortable position and try to nap. The napping was an effort in futility, as I'd known it would be. My mind raced a mile a minute; the harder I tried to relax, the faster it churned, flitting from one thought to another.

After ten or fifteen minutes, she interrupted my thoughts to say, "Your body is relaxed, but you are not sleeping. I'm going to give you something to help you sleep."

"A sleeping pill will put me out pretty fast," I said.

"It's not a sleeping pill. Have you ever taken Dramamine?"

"For motion sickness?" I asked. "I didn't know it was a sleeping pill."

"It will help you relax. It's not absolutely necessary that you sleep," she said, "but if you are able to sleep, it will speed up the test."

She gave me two Dramamine tablets. While they were taking effect, she decided to perform two other tests.

The first involved blinking lights. She tested me twice: once with my eyes open and again with them closed.

"Just look at the light," she instructed. "It's quite bright. It will blink slowly, at first; then more rapidly. You can blink, but try to keep your head still. Don't wrinkle your forehead or grit your teeth."

A simple test, but when the light went into its rapid-blink mode, I was reminded of psychological torture and knew I would be unable to handle this kind of treatment for any length of time without going berserk. When my eyes were open, the speed of the blinking light seemed to reach a plateau after a certain time, and the speed didn't increase. But when the test was administered with my eyes closed, the speed of the blinking lights seemed to increase in rapidity every time. I watched a kaleidoscope of light changes flash before my eyes.

The second test was a breathing test.

"I want you to breathe deeply with your mouth open. Breathe as fast as you can for three minutes. I want you to really huff and puff," she explained,

The test sounded simple enough as I began the deep-breathing exercise. After a minute and a half, I was certain I would pass out or go flying off into space. I was so lightheaded I felt I could float and was fearful that I might just do that, or instead, roll off the bed and drop onto the floor. I slowed my breathing slightly to regain equilibrium.

"Keep on breathing," she coaxed. "You only have a minute and a half to go." I kept on huffing, but I knew I had slowed the pace considerably, putting longer pauses between each breath as I attempted to regain control of my body. At the end of three minutes, the test was over, but I had lost control of my body. It shook with convulsions and shivered and trembled uncontrollably. I knew I experienced a form of hyperventilation caused by over-oxygenating the body.

"I thought I would pass out," I commented, still trying to regain control.

"You're experiencing a normal reaction," the technician advised. "No one has passed out on me yet."

Small consolation, I thought as the time between convulsions lengthened. After several more minutes, my body calmed. With the convulsions almost stopped, she encouraged me to lie on my side.

"Try to sleep."

First they get me all hyped up, I thought, *and now they tell me to sleep.* I felt more wide awake than ever. While I didn't consciously fight sleep, the harder I tried to relax, the more wide awake I became.

The technician adjusted an electrode on my left side, the side I lay on, and suggested I try to sleep on my back. By now, I had stopped convulsing.

"Can I have something to block the light from the EEG machine?"

She handed me a towel to cover my eyes. While it blocked the light, it didn't block my thoughts. My mind continued to race—a full-blown case of insomnia. I should have scheduled the test for late afternoon. Maybe then I would have been more tired.

Time crept by slowly. Finally, I asked if I could return to my side. The pressure in the back of my head had become uncomfortable. With her permission, I turned to my left side.

Following the hyperventilation test, I noticed the spinning sensation increased each time I moved my head to change positions. Now, lying on my left side, I finally relaxed, and my mind slowed. At one point I felt very close to sleep, although I never quite drifted off.

The EEG took about an hour. Attaching and detaching the electrodes increased the time to an hour and a half. Although the last test was painless, as I got up to leave I noticed the pressure inside my head was building, and the vertigo had returned.

I commented aloud to myself, "MS, June."

"MS?" the technician repeated.

"Move slow," I replied, explaining Bud's comment and then adding, "I thought Dramamine was supposed to *control* motion sickness, not make it *worse*."

Following the EEG test, I decided the source of my problem was in my head, not in my hormones.

Saturday, November 20, 1982

The vertigo was worse than ever last night, aggravated, no doubt, by the EEG testing. But when I awoke this morning, I felt clear-headed. My only discomfort was intense chest pain on the right side. It lasted only a short time after arising. As the day progressed, I felt more clear-headed than I have for weeks, as if the hyperventilation had reoxygenated my brain.

I knew I needed to learn more about vitamin B6 and why I needed to take it. I started reading Adelle Davis's book *Let's Eat Right to Keep Fit*,[13] which my friend Harriet Hammon had given me.

"Keep whichever books you want and give the rest to the church book sale," Harriet had said, and for some reason, I had kept this one about vitamin deficiencies.

"If you take one or more B vitamins, you increase your need for all the other vitamins in the B group," Davis contended. "The increased need for the ones you do not take may cause you to develop deficiencies of them; these deficiencies can cause far more harm than the vitamins which you take can do good."[14]

Now I wondered if the B12 shots had caused me to develop deficiencies in some of the other B vitamins and were now resulting in my current neurological problems. Perhaps the B6 I took for hormonal imbalance added to the deficiencies, causing a B vitamin imbalance. I decided to experiment by taking brewer's yeast every day. Brewer's yeast, according to Davis, contained all the B vitamins naturally and in balanced proportions. If I was deficient, the yeast should restore B vitamin balance.

On November 21, 1982, I started taking two teaspoons of brewer's yeast, blended together in "tiger's milk" for breakfast. Davis said there were a number of formulas for tiger's milk, using different fruits and

---

[13] Adelle Davis, AB, MS. *Let's Eat Right to Keep Fit* (New York: Harcourt, Brace and Company, 1954).

[14] Ibid., 118.

fruit juices. Each person should find one they enjoyed. The one I found most palatable was 6 ounces of milk, 6 ounces of orange or other fruit juice, and half a banana, blended together with two teaspoons of brewer's yeast.

Monday, November 22, 1982

Following several relatively clear-headed days, I felt more energized this morning, but the old familiar nausea washed over me at lunchtime. The back of my head ached again with pressure. This morning I woke with a small headache but had mentally suppressed it. *How long have I been practicing this mind-over-matter control?* I wondered.

I felt hot, but when I took my temperature, it was normal. Hyperthyroidism (thyroid overdose), I knew, could cause feelings of warmth, but so could hot flashes from menopause. *Am I still overdosed on thyroid?* I wondered. And if I was, what permanent damage could it wreak on my system? An overactive thyroid, I had learned, could also cause eye problems.

After lunch, the nausea passed. *Hypoglycemia?* I only had tiger's milk for breakfast. Maybe it wasn't enough. My head felt ready to explode, so I lay down for half an hour. Lying down always helped.

At seven o'clock that evening, Dr. Johnson called to report that my EEG was normal.

"What do we do now?" I asked.

"I'm not sure," he replied. "I don't have your file handy. I'll have to call you back tomorrow."

CHAPTER 25

THE FIFTY-THOUSAND-PIECE PUZZLE

Tuesday, November 23, 1982
I am still reading Adelle Davis's book *Let's Eat Right to Keep Fit*, along with other information from the public library about B vitamins. I'm convinced my problem is an acute B vitamin deficiency.

I first experienced the mental dullness and fuzziness after taking the B12 shots. Davis contends, "The action of all B vitamins is synergistic [meaning they act together with each other]. One alone or several together increase the need for the B vitamins not supplied" (p. 100). Overdosing on one B vitamin causes an imbalance in the ones not supplied.

Under Betty's care, I had taken estrogen for more than a year without the addition of B6. When I first noticed the mental dullness, my body undoubtedly had become deficient in B6. The B12 shots may have multiplied the symptoms of the B6 deficiency.

Furthermore, Davis claimed a B1 deficiency caused digestive disturbances, including hard, dry stools and symptoms that mimic hypoglycemia. I'd had both problems for years. Maybe that explained the severe hypoglycemic attack experienced at convention last year, followed by the mini-hypoglycemic reactions afterwards.

A deficiency of niacin, another B vitamin, can cause a variety of symptoms, including a coated tongue, flattened mushroom-type taste buds, and deep crevices down the center of the tongue.

I rushed to the bathroom mirror to check my tongue. It was white and fuzzy-looking, as usual. I had often mentioned this fact to Betty because as a little girl, Mom told us "a coated tongue means you are sick." Betty always dismissed my concerns as of no consequence. Now I noticed the deep ridges in my tongue and the tiny, flat, mushroom-like shapes on the back of my tongue.

I hurried to the living room where Bud was sitting.

"Stick out your tongue," I ordered. He complied. His tongue was evenly red with neither ridges nor mushrooms.

According to Davis, niacin deficiencies could cause canker sores and cheek ulcers. I'd been plagued with both much of my life. When the stomach fails to produce enough hydrochloric acid for the proper absorption of calcium and iron, nervous disorders and anemia occur. When digestion is faulty, gas and flatulence occur. Constipation is often an early symptom. In years past, severe gas pains had bothered me so much I had entirely quit drinking carbonated beverages.

"Persons undersupplied with niacin often suffer feelings of strain and tension, stress, insomnia, dizziness, nervousness, irritability, and frequent recurring headaches," Davis wrote. "If the deficiency is allowed to become more severe, mental dullness, depression, hostility and suspicion may grow in intensity. Sometimes a person feels like crying frequently without knowing what he is crying about" (p. 92). She had described my symptoms perfectly.

"Niacin is a vitamin which can be made in the body from the amino acid, tryptophan, provided adequate protein and other B vitamins are generously supplied. It is known that an enzyme containing B6 (deaminase) is necessary for the conversion of tryptophan to niacin," she stated on page 93. *Bingo*, I thought. *That's me.*

I learned that women on contraceptive pills or female hormones containing estrogen need more B6 in their daily diets, as do most women (and some men) over age sixty.

The theory seemed to confirm the reason I immediately began to feel better after Dr. Lance added B6 to my diet. Thinking back, I realized the dizziness had recurred when I allowed my B6 level to drop back to 50 milligrams a day. Apparently, I needed the higher 100 milligrams or 200 milligrams dosage.

Davis pointed out that liver, brewer's yeast, and wheat germ were among the best sources of complete B vitamins—products most people seldom eat, certainly not on a daily basis. Brewer's yeast, she cautioned, should be taken in small amounts at first—one or two teaspoons a day—especially if digestion is very faulty. Otherwise, so much gas will be produced that the intestinal tract will "balloon." However, as the B vitamin deficiency is corrected, and the yeast is more completely digested, gas and the resultant feeling of fullness will disappear.

When Dr. Johnson called later that day, he suggested that I should next see an ear, nose, and throat specialist for an ENG (electronystagmogram) to check the workings of the inner ear. An ENG, I learned, checks the muscles that control eye movements; checks how well the eyes, inner ears, and brain help you keep your balance; and checks for damage to the nerves that may cause dizziness, vertigo, and loss of balance.

"I think I have a massive B vitamin deficiency," I said, explaining my theory. "Have you heard of it?"

He admitted he had not.

"Is it necessary for me to have the ENG right away?"

"No," he replied. "Try your theory for a month and then let me know the results. We can do the ENG later. If your theory works, maybe you ought to write a paper."

I wondered if he was being facetious or serious.

I hung up, reassured. I had found another doctor open to suggestions, not close-minded about vitamin deficiencies or their consequences, as some doctors are. He was a doctor not afraid to let his patient help with her recovery.

Next day, Fran Forrester, our across-the-street neighbor, stopped to visit. Four years earlier she had recovered from lung cancer surgery. Recently, she had undergone two days of testing for vertigo at Mercy Hospital. The diagnosis was niacin deficiency; the treatment was nicotinic acid.

Some days I felt like someone had thrown a fifty-thousand-piece jigsaw puzzle at me, with the admonition to find all the pieces and put the puzzle back together again. Bit by bit, I was finding the pieces, and they were starting to fit together. Someday soon, I hoped to see the entire picture—*clearly*.

CHAPTER 26

THE MYSTERY DEEPENS

Thursday, December 9, 1982

I called Dr. Fields's office and talked to his receptionist.

"Do you know if there is a test to check the level of B vitamins in my body?" I gave her a quick rundown of my B vitamin deficiency theory. Although she asked me to repeat the information so she could write it down, she sounded skeptical. I didn't blame her.

The only way I could determine whether my symptoms were caused by hormonal or B vitamin depletion was to make a list of all my symptoms and the corresponding B vitamin deficiencies that could cause them.

At Dr. Lance's suggestion, I had increased the estrogen level to 0.625 milligrams. The headaches and pressure in the back of my head disappeared a few days later.

As I completed more research on vitamin B deficiencies, I wondered if they could also cause learning disabilities. When my symptoms were most severe, I felt learning disabled—like my mind could absorb only so much information and no more. I likened it to an overloaded computer memory bank that, when it reached saturation, caused the brain cells to slow down and/or shut off.

The summer my eleven-year-old nephew, Jimmy, lived with us, he had been termed "learning disabled." He had come to Arizona so I could work with him, using the Laubach reading method of phonics.

In the 1970s, I had used the Laubach teaching method while helping Vietnamese immigrant children learn English and hoped to help Jimmy overcome his reading difficulties by working with him daily on a one-to-one basis. The new "sight method of reading" being used at his school had not taught him how to sound out words phonetically. We worked on his reading for a couple hours each morning. He'd read the lesson aloud to me so I could tell where he was having difficulty. Sometimes his mind seemed to reach a plateau of learning, after which he seemed unable to assimilate further information. Usually, I could tell when he reached that point by the way he stumbled over simple words.

"Do you feel like your mind is a computer, and your memory banks are overloaded?" I would question him.

If he replied, "yes," we would take a short break before returning to the task of reading. Now I wondered if brewer's yeast could have improved his retention ability and lengthened his attention span. Like me, Jimmy suffered periodically from canker sores. Did he also have B vitamin deficiencies?

Still, if there was such a simple connection between B vitamin deficiencies and learning disabilities, why hadn't someone already discovered it?

Later that evening, Dr. Fields returned my call.

"Is there a test you can give me to check the B vitamin levels in my body to see if they are in balance?" I asked.

He said there was none.

"I think I have a massive B vitamin deficiency," I explained.

"Why do you think that?"

"I've been reading a book by Adelle Davis, the nutritionist. She says a coated tongue with deep fissures is indicative of a total B vitamin deficiency."

He listened patiently and then said, "Yours isn't all *that coated.*"

"My husband's isn't coated at all."

"All tongues are different."

"But she also says"—I reached for the book that I had conveniently placed near the telephone—"that the action of all B vitamins is *synergistic*." I opened the book and read, "'One alone or several together increase the need for the B vitamins not supplied. Deficiencies of the undersupplied vitamins may produce abnormalities which can do more harm than the vitamins obtained can do good.' I started having these severe mental blip-outs after taking the B12 shots last year. I think my system was depleted of all B vitamins—or at least it was thrown out of balance."

"B vitamins are replaced in your system daily from the foods you eat," Dr. Fields stated.

"I charted a list of all my symptoms and the B vitamin deficiencies they represent. It seems to indicate a deficiency of all—or almost all—B vitamins. I know I've been deficient in vitamin B6. When I called Dr. Lance's office about the nausea and dizziness, he increased my B6 dosage to 200 milligrams a day—and it helped. It's a proven fact that women taking female hormones, even birth control pills, need extra B6."

"You shouldn't need more than 50 milligrams of B6 a day," he said, thoughtfully, almost as if talking to himself.

"Fifty is what I took when the dizziness started," I explained. "I need 200 milligrams a day. After I started taking 200 milligrams a day, my dizziness disappeared. It acted like a tranquilizer for me. I've had symptoms of B vitamin deficiencies for years. They are just getting more severe." I needed to convince him, but how? "For years I've had chapped lips, symptomatic of a B2 deficiency. Whenever I pointed this out to Betty, her standard recommendation was, 'Drink more water.' According to Adelle Davis, excess water just washes more of the B vitamins out of your system—"

"You don't have the chapped lips of a severe deficiency," he interrupted. "That is usually seen only in countries suffering serious malnutrition. You don't look malnourished."

"I'm not," I agreed, "but all the B vitamins are found in quantity only in foods such as brewer's yeast, wheat germ, or liver—foods most people seldom if ever eat and certainly not daily."

"You get B vitamins in *other* foods."

"But I think *my* B vitamins are out of sync or else my body isn't utilizing them properly. Brewer's yeast is balanced, and it seems to be helping."

"It won't hurt you," he reluctantly conceded, implying it wouldn't help either.

"I also read that thyroid overdose can deplete your system of B vitamins."

"That's true," he agreed. I almost fainted to hear him make an affirmative comment. "What are you taking now?"

"One grain a day," I said. "Remember, we reduced it from two grains the last time I was in, but I may *still* be overdosed."

"Why don't you come in, and we'll check it again," he suggested.

"When should I come?" I asked. "Last time you said you'd recheck it in three months—at my next visit. Can you tell if there's been a change in just two months?"

"Make an appointment in about a week," he instructed.

From my reading, I knew changes in thyroid medications were not immediately evident. Sometimes it took a full three weeks for a thyroid pill to effect change.

The puzzle pieces were beginning to fit together. Since reducing my thyroid dosage in mid-October, I had changed from my usual insomniac self. Now, I fell into a deep, fatigued, almost drugged sleep. Furthermore, my body didn't feel like it was racing in high gear all the time. *How long*, I wondered, *have I been pepped up with thyroid medicine?* I had taken thyroid drugs for years. In the summer of 1981, Betty had increased the dosage from one grain to two because I continued to complain about feeling fatigued. The summer of the iron and B12 shots—the summer of the great fatigue.

Were we at last reaching the end of the road—an answer to my health problems? Could the thyroid overdose be wreaking permanent health problems on my body? A new concern? Or had we identified the problem in time to prevent permanent, serious damage? More and more unanswered questions remained to be resolved.

I thanked Dr. Fields and hung up the phone, wondering if I sounded like a stark raving maniac. But exhilaration overcame me now because of his response. He hadn't laughed or openly rejected my theory. He had listened—with understanding—and finally with some agreement.

God was leading me to the right diagnosis; I was convinced of it. Just as He had led me to this right doctor, a healer in the truest sense of the word.

Another week would give me more time to research my B vitamin theory and give Dr. Fields, perhaps, the same opportunity. At our next meeting, I planned to confront him with evidence in hand.

Later, as I mulled over our conversation, I decided that what Dr. Fields attempted to tell me, in his own nebulous way, was that if my system had become depleted of B vitamins from a B12 overdose a year ago, by now my body should have replaced the vitamins through natural nutrition. If the vitamins were still depleted or were not being replaced, something else must be the cause. Something, perhaps, like thyroid overdose.

A week later, blood was drawn for another T4 thyroid test, but I did not have an appointment to see Dr. Fields that day.

Wednesday, December 22, 1982

Dr. Fields called this morning with the results of my thyroid test—it was 5.4, about a point lower but still within a normal range.

"If you start feeling fatigued," he counseled, "you might want to raise it again to two milligrams a day."

"Milligrams?" I questioned. "Is that the same as a grain?"

"Yes."

"My body doesn't feel like it's racing all the time anymore," I reported. "I'm sleeping better."

"Then stick with the dosage you are taking."

"Adrenal dysfunction," I said, "can cause some of the symptoms I've experienced. Is there a way to measure if the adrenal glands are working properly?"

"Yes," he said, "there is a test to measure blood cortisone levels."

"Do you recommend it for me?"

"You don't really have symptoms of adrenal dysfunction," he stated. "Your blood pressure is normal. Your sodium and potassium levels are normal. The sodium/potassium levels usually show some abnormalities with an adrenal problem."

"I am feeling better overall," I admitted. "I guess the thing to do is to continue the brewer's yeast and come in next month for my regular blood work."

He agreed that was the best course of action for the time being.

Now I was confused. Nothing seemed to make sense except that I had a massive Vitamin B deficiency *that couldn't be proved.*

On December 28, about a month after beginning the brewer's yeast, I wrote a four-page progress report reiterating my B vitamin deficiency theory to Dr. Johnson, the neurologist, and sent copies of the letter to both Dr. Fields and Dr. Lance.

CHAPTER 27

"IT COULD BE MELANOMA"

At my next appointment with Dr. Fields, on January 10, 1983, he greeted me as he entered the examining room, "So … you think you've cured yourself." He had read his copy of the letter I'd written to Dr. Johnson.

"I don't know," I answered, not knowing exactly how to react to his comment. "I hope so. That's what I want *you* to tell me."

"How are you feeling?"

"Better than I have felt in years," I acknowledged. "I feel like I have regained my brain." Then I said, "You mentioned on the phone that I might need some B vitamin supplements. How would you know which ones or how much of each to prescribe?"

He shook his head. "We wouldn't. It's pretty much trial and error. But you say you are feeling fine. If I were you, I wouldn't change anything you are doing."

"The brewer's yeast is a little inconvenient to carry with me all the time," I murmured, "especially if I'm traveling and can't be home in the afternoons to take it when I get the seizures."

"There are worse things," he sympathized, although he didn't elaborate on what they might be. Nor did I ask. "Sometimes we have to live with the little inconveniences in our lives," he said, letting me know he didn't intend to prescribe any B vitamins to replace the yeast in my diet. "And what did you say was in the yeast?" he asked abruptly.

"All the B vitamins," I replied, "in a balanced ratio."

It was a short visit. He checked my heart, lungs, and lymph glands. Everything seemed normal, but he still wanted to see me again in three months. Although feeling better, I still was not totally well.

On April 15, 1983, I had my next three-month checkup with Dr. Fields.

"I have lots of questions," I said in greeting.

He smiled, nodded, sat down, and waited for me to begin.

"Do I have pyridoxine deficiency anemia?"

"The bone marrow test didn't indicate that you did," he replied, flipping backward through the pages of my file to the bone marrow results.

"Pyridoxine deficient anemia responds only to 200 milligrams of B6 daily," I said, plunging ahead. "That was when I started to feel better, when I began taking the higher dose of B6."

"You might have had a B vitamin deficiency caused by thyroid overdose or some other imbalance," he conceded.

"B6 deficiency causes a breakdown of the myelin sheath of the nerve endings," I continued. "I am wondering if I might have been in the early stages of multiple sclerosis."

"I don't think so—"

"Hear me out," I interrupted. "I have or have had symptoms associated with multiple sclerosis: dizziness accompanied by nausea and vomiting; fatigue and weakness; pain from neuritis (my leg pain); disturbed sleep patterns; and sensitivity to cold. I've always been a "freezy" person. Surgical operations contribute to flare-ups, as do rage, anxiety, and fear, as well as forgetfulness and disruption of rapid recall from brain seizures that resemble epilepsy. I still have these occasionally but never have had the muscle spasms, tremors, or jerking.

"Paging back through my diary, I discovered that the many severe spells of dizziness and fuzziness occurred after I treated myself for sinus congestion with antihistamines that Betty recommended. MS is treated with histamines—just the opposite of what I was taking."

"MS is very hard to diagnose," he said. "Did your neurologist find any abnormalities?'

"He said everything was normal."

"I don't think you have MS. I hope you don't have MS. But if you do, the symptoms will recur."

"Could MS cause the high sed rate? Would the demylination process cause that?"

"Your sed rate isn't excessively high. A cold could cause it to be that high."

"Well, I'm still getting these spots of blood under my toenails."

"Can I see?" he asked, his question a mixture of curiosity and interest.

I removed my sock.

"How long have you had this?"

"A couple of months. I think I noticed them again around Christmas. You remember both toenails were purple when I saw you in October 1981. When the toenails grew out, about a year later, it went away. Now it's coming back again but only in one toenail. At first it was only one tiny spot; then as the toenail grew out a little, another spot appeared just below it."

"It could be a melanoma," he said thoughtfully. "I'd like you to see a surgeon and have it checked. It may be nothing, but melanomas are sometimes very hard to detect."

I showed him the Arcadia Clinic bulletin I had brought with me, featuring atomidine—the thyroid medicine I first received while under their care.

"This is what I took before they started me on prescription thyroid medicine," I said. "According to this article, it's radioactive iodine."

"It wasn't radioactive iodine," he broke in. "They wouldn't have been able to get radioactive iodine."

"Could it have caused the thyroid to speed up or slow down?" I asked.

He shrugged his shoulders. "I have no idea."

"Could the endometriosis have caused a hormonal imbalance that might have caused the B6 depletion?"

"I don't know that either," he admitted.

Down to the last item on my list, I said, "A 1974 *Journal of the American Medical Association*[15] article stated that 500 milligrams of vitamin C can destroy 95 percent of the vitamin B12 in a meal. Is that true?"

"I'd like to see that article," he responded with interest.

"My reference notes are at home," I replied, "but I'll look it up and give you the exact issue number."

"I would appreciate that. If it's true, it could have long-range effects."

"Yes," I agreed. "People may be causing their own symptoms of stress by overdosing themselves on vitamin C, depleting their systems of vitamin B12, and throwing all the other B vitamins out of balance." It was a theory I had considered before, but I wanted the confirmation of a medical expert.

My lab work that day consisted of tests for hemoglobin, sedimentation rate, platelet count, urinalysis, chem-16 profile, and T4 thyroid test. All the tests came back normal. The hemoglobin was a healthy 13.7; the sed rate had dropped from 40 to 27; the white cell count of 4.9 was slightly low but okay; and the thyroid of 6.0 was up slightly but still in a normal range. My blood pressure was a normal 128/70. Dr. Fields still listed "chronic anemia" for my diagnosis.

At home, I checked my reference notes for the *JAMA* article. After lunch I found the issue at the public library, copied it, and left the copy at Dr. Fields's office. Rereading the article, I learned that not only was vitamin C hazardous to B12, but overdoses of iron might also deplete the system of vitamin B12.

In some ways, I felt like I'd been on a witch hunt, trying to find and exorcise all the demons within my body. As I learned more about holistic

---

[15] Victor Herbert, MD, and Elizabeth Jacob, MD. "Destruction of Vitamin B12 by Ascorbic Acid," *Journal of the American Medical Association*, October 14, 1974. 241–42.

medicine and its connection to occultism in the New Age movement, I wondered if an exorcism was what I *really* needed. (But I never resorted to this extreme practice.)

Another Easter passed. The following Wednesday, April 20, 1983, I met with Dr. Switzer, the surgeon scheduled to remove my toenail.

He said, "It looks like a hematoma [blood clot] rather than a melanoma [cancer]. The toenail will be removed on Friday and biopsied. If malignant cells are found, the toe also will be removed."

I decided not to tell anyone about this impending surgery, but Phyllis called that night with the prayer chain. At the end of the list, she asked, "And how are *you* doing?"

I felt that many of my friends were tired of hearing about my never-ending bout with the possibility of cancer. So was I. I didn't want to be labeled a hypochondriac, nor did I want to receive false pity, but all of a sudden I began telling her about my upcoming surgery.

"Oh, my goodness," she said with genuine concern. "We need to put *you* on the prayer chain too."

"Yes, I suppose so," I answered, not because I was afraid of the surgery or what they might find, but because I had come to covet the extra prayers I knew would be raised to God by fellow believers. I had come to believe and accept the real power of corporate prayer. *Please, God, don't let it be cancer.*

On April 22, 1983, I arrived on the third floor of the surgicenter at eight o'clock in the morning, feeling very calm. It surprised me that I had to disrobe and don a paper hospital gown. I expected only to have to remove my shoe and sock to have the surgery performed. The sterile precautions, I assumed, were to keep germs to a minimum. My foot was liberally bathed with an iodine solution, and Novocain was injected to dull the pain. The toenail was removed in a pie-shaped slice. I had brought along a magazine and read while the doctor and his nurse worked on my toe.

"It's in the toenail," the doctor exclaimed when he removed the piece.

"The hematoma is in the toenail?" I asked.

"It's not a hematoma," he replied. "It's not even in the toe."

Afterward, he assured me he was almost 100 percent certain there was no danger of melanoma. Although numbed, I could walk on my foot and was released to go home about ten o'clock. The Novocain wore off about four that afternoon. Pain was minimal. Although I had been given a prescription for pain meds, I didn't need any. The next day, I removed the large bandage, replaced it with a Band-Aid, and was able to wear my shoe again.

On Thursday, April 28, when I called for the results of the biopsy, the nurse who took my call said, "From the report, it looks like the biopsy hadn't been taken deep enough. More tissue might be needed."

I didn't relish the thought of giving "another pound of flesh" and visualized them removing the toe, then the leg at the knee to cure the shin pain, then removing the thigh to excise the hip pain. Then what? How much higher could they go without cutting into vital organs? No, I decided, I would not let them chop away at my body. *How quickly my trust in God had vanished.*

On May 3, I met with Dr. Switzer for my postsurgical checkup. "Everything looks fine," he said.

"You mean I don't need more surgery?" I asked.

"Where did you get that idea?

I explained my Thursday conversation with his office nurse. He waited a few minutes for me to put on my sock and shoe before we marched out to the front desk.

"Who told Mrs. Schmidt her test results?"

A young woman stepped forward. "I did."

"She has been put through unnecessary worry," he said. "What did you tell her?"

The girl explained that because he was out of the office, unavailable for consultation, she had taken the report to another doctor in their office. That doctor had interpreted it to mean additional tissue might still be needed. "I only told her what he told me," she said.

"I never suspected anything," Dr. Switzer explained, "so I only sent a few surface cells. Nothing was found in them, as this report confirms, but I didn't expect them to find anything, as I told you after we did the surgery." He turned to me. "Don't worry about it; there is nothing to be concerned about."

Relieved and reassured by the manner in which he had confronted and resolved the situation, I thanked him, shook his hand, and left, happy now that I didn't have to worry about losing my big toe—or anything else.

Bud and I had been referred to a medical malpractice lawyer. After talking with him, we learned that if you live and recover, you have no basis for a medical malpractice suit. Unless permanent damage can be determined within three years of treatment, no reputable lawyer will take your lawsuit. If there is no provable cause for dollar damages, no lawyer would take a medical malpractice suit that would not enrich him.

"Let me get this straight," I said. "In order to put my holistic practitioners out of business, I would have had to *die*?" Then I quickly added, "I don't think I'm quite ready to make that kind of sacrifice just to rid the world of holistic medicine."

I felt my holistic medical doctors had robbed me of some of the most productive years of my life. They had possibly cost us the chance to become parents. They had caused me to undergo untold unnecessary tests, including many radioactive ones and other procedures in our quest to find the root cause and cure for my symptoms, many of which they had created. For months my mind had drifted in and out of a drug-induced haze not of my own making. And yet, I couldn't sue them out of business.

Conversely, I felt relieved when I learned no lawyer would take our case. Did I want to endure the stress of a jury trial? No. And now I wouldn't have to worry that anything I wrote and published exposing their ungodly practices would damage or interfere with an upcoming lawsuit. I decided that, with God's help, I would *write* holistic medicine out of business.

CHAPTER 28

HEALED: BODY, MIND, AND SPIRIT

Between the time I had the meltdown after returning from our vacation trip in July 1982 and when I visited Dr. Fields in October 1982, I had become so frustrated with the lack of progress in discovering the origin of my illness or how to treat it that one day I just stood in the middle of our living room, lifted my hands heavenward, and cried aloud to the empty space, "God, I just want to be *whole* again!"

And God, who listens to his wayward children and is faithful, answered my desperate plea for healing. From that moment, I began to see progress in my recovery. I continued to badger Dr. Fields, believing that I never needed the thyroid medicine prescribed by my holistic doctors. Dr. Fields reluctantly but gradually halved my thyroid doses, until three years later, completely off all thyroid medication, I felt normal again.

My T4 readings remained in a normal range *every time* we tested them after each reduction. Although at first he was hesitant to decrease my dose of thyroid medication, Dr. Fields soon began to see a pattern and continued to work with me. Once I was weaned off all thyroid medicine, Dr. Fields finally said, "I don't think you need the brewer's yeast anymore either."

The yeast had become part of my daily diet. I took about a half cup of yeast daily, equally divided between morning and afternoon doses. I was afraid that once I stopped, all the horrible symptoms would return, and I would have a total breakdown—mental, physical, and emotional. Eventually, however, I did stop, and the symptoms didn't return.

I theorized that my holistic doctors, by gradually increasing the thyroid medication when my T4 readings registered in a normal range, had caused my body to build up a tolerance to the higher dose. Thus, subsequent T4 readings continued to register in a normal range. And yet the overdose quantities put into my body were affecting and breaking down my whole system. If I hadn't discovered and told Dr. Fields that my T4 reading was 6.0 when Betty increased my dosage by a whole grain, who knows how long I would have continued down this destructive pathway?

Once completely off all thyroid medication, my T4 readings remained in a normal range. Dr. Fields admitted he had never before encountered such a thing happening.

I still wonder if my holistic practitioners *knew* they were creating a massive vitamin B deficiency in my body and had deliberately made me sick with their overdoses of thyroid medication, thinking no one would ever figure it out—and I would *never* get well. Some doctors know just enough medicine to make their patients sick—*and keep them sick*—to gain long-term-care patients. Or was this overdose an accidental result of their unprofessional medical practices? They had to know they weren't following standard medical procedures when they continued to increase my thyroid medicine dosage, even when all my test results showed my thyroid levels were within normal ranges. Were they, in fact, setting me up for later-life thyroid problems? I'll never know that for certain.

Almost thirty years later, on November 22, 2011, after being diagnosed with *multinodular Hashimoto's thyroiditis*, my left thyroid gland was removed. So many nodules had grown on it that it was deviating and displacing my trachea and esophagus. The gland had grown to about the size of a fist and soon would have affected my ability to swallow.

Discovered accidentally during a chest CT scan for another condition, my endocrinologist immediately suspected cancer, explaining, "You have so many nodules growing on your left thyroid gland that I can't even biopsy it. I wouldn't know where to begin." She recommended we go right to surgery. Once again, I faced the possibility of cancer. But, secure in God's faithfulness, I went into surgery unafraid, surrounded again by prayer warriors. Whatever the outcome, I knew it would be okay. I was at peace with my mortality. It was a good place to be.

There was no cancer, but I'll always wonder if this surgery was necessitated by the previous thyroid overdose.

After losing my left thyroid gland I was again placed on thyroid medication—75 *micro*grams, a far cry from the 200 *milli*grams my holistic practitioner prescribed when I had both thyroid glands intact and functioning normally. My current dosage is more than twenty-six times *less* than the amount I took while under Betty Miller's holistic health care.

Because I was back on thyroid medicine, I returned to taking brewer's yeast again, two heaping teaspoons a day in my morning juice. Perhaps it is a placebo effect, but I do feel better when taking it.

The problems within our church also were brought to a conclusion. At the annual meeting in January 1983, I stood up and said, "Before this meeting is over, I hope someone addresses this concern: Last year we had over one thousand *inactive* members—about a third of our membership. This year we've lost another four hundred members to inactivity—back-door losses. What is being done to stem this flow?" The room became very quiet as if everyone was stunned. I continued. "Our church has hosted an evangelism conference two years in a row, but *we* don't even have an active, functioning evangelism committee ourselves." I sat down.

Later, I learned that when the meeting concluded, fifteen members came forward to serve on an evangelism committee. Apparently, I wasn't the only person concerned about the direction in which our church was—or was not—heading.

Two days later, I received an anonymous letter in the mail. Enclosed was a column from Sunday's newspaper, titled "Self-acceptance key to destructive behavior." Someone, not happy with my comments at Sunday's meeting, apparently thought I was displaying destructive behavior and wanted to cast aspersions on my character, but who didn't have the gumption or grace to reveal his or her own identity.

That same week, the president of the congregation and the assistant pastor visited Bud and me in our home, revealing that our senior pastor thought I was "out to get him."

"That's preposterous," I replied, shocked that he would even think that I harbored a vendetta against him. "If that's the way he feels, we can solve that problem in a hurry." I was hurt and angry. "We will leave the church." And we did. Not only did we leave the church, but we joined a church in a different synod. And because we left the synod, I could no longer continue as *The Communicator* editor.

I boxed all my *Communicator* files for the next editor. Unexpected and unrestrained tears rolled down my cheeks as I worked, almost like the day nine months earlier when I'd lost control, except today I knew *why* I was crying. I was losing another piece of my life. The newsletter had become an integral part of me; I was losing my creative expression.

But God had other plans for me. A door was closing, but a window was opening. I joined a Christian writers group, determined to expose the fraud of holistic medicine. And in the ensuing years, I found I had other stories to write.

But I received one more anonymous letter. In March 1983, an article from *A New Heart* magazine, published by Hospital Christian Fellowship, arrived in my mail. The article enclosed was "Holistic Medicine: What Is It? What Is It Not?" by Aubrey Beauchamp, RN. All the rage and anger I still harbored toward my holistic practitioners was rekindled. Because I didn't know who had sent the article, I didn't know whether the author was speaking for or against holistic medicine, and I felt betrayed all over again.

Finally, after seething for several days, I summoned the courage to actually read the article. Then I knew it had been sent by a friend concerned about the influence holistic medicine still held over my life. The article's author concluded, "I firmly believe that holistic medicine, as well as any other branch of the healing profession, in order to be effective *must* be based on Christian principles." Our holistic doctor who, early in our medical relationship, suggested we have our astrology charts cast clearly displayed he was *not* a Christian. Christians don't believe in or practice astrology. But my husband and I didn't realize that fact at the time.

The article further stated that the holistic medical movement was rooted in Eastern occult and metaphysical practices. It spoke about a group called Spiritual Counterfeits Project, who sought to expose holistic medicine and other false spiritual practices. Later, I became acquainted with the National Council Against Health Fraud. The two organizations opened my eyes to other deceitful practices carried out in the name of holy medicine.

In time, I learned that Dorothy Dorring, my friend from our church women's group, who had ministered to me during my recovery and whose judgment and opinions I respected, had requested that the editor of *The New Heart* magazine send the article to me. I only wish it hadn't been sent anonymously. I never learned who sent the other anonymous letter.

On December 24, 1982, I received a response to my complaint to the Arizona Board of Medical Examiners that said, in part,

> The Board determined in Open Session that inappropriate evaluation of your health care needs resulted in inadequate care. Accordingly the Board determined to file this matter with a letter of concern to Dr. Berry. Specifically, the Board was concerned about the inadequate evaluation for anemia and the doctor's authorization to allow the illegal use of pre-signed prescriptions by his nurse practitioner. The Board also noted its concern that there may not be necessary direction and supervision of the nurse practitioner by Dr. Berry.

In the medical community, I'd heard that a letter of concern was considered a serious punishment, but to me, it seemed like a slap on the wrist. I was so disappointed. Because I didn't know about the thyroid overdose when I wrote the letter of complaint, it hadn't been included. Now I wondered if it would even have made a difference.

The following February 8, 1983, I called the County Medical Society's Referral Service, asking if they referred patients to Arcadia Clinic. The person who answered replied, "We do not. They are considered a naturopathic clinic. Do you want to be referred to the Naturopathic Association?"

"I do *not*," I replied, thinking that at least I accomplished one thing—unsuspecting patients would no longer be referred to the Doctors Berry by the County Medical Society, as I had been.

Instead of keeping my body in balance, as they had promised to do when I first visited their clinic, my holistic doctors had succeeded in putting my body out of balance, resulting in far-reaching medical consequences, proving their brand of medicine was neither holy nor healthy.

Through follow-up letters with the Arizona Board of Medical Examiners, I learned Dr. Jim had received a second letter of concern, and Dr. Mary had also received a letter of concern. Yet they still continued to practice medicine.

Do I *hate* my holistic doctors for what they did to me? No. Did I forgive them for their mistreatment? Yes. While they attempted to steal my body and my mind, I was determined that they would not steal my soul. Hate does not affect the person being hated. The person may not even know he or she is hated. But hate, like a cancer, will eat *you* up and eventually destroy *you*. I refused to give them that kind of power and control over my life.

On the other hand, I refused to ignore what they did to me and continued to do to other unsuspecting patients with their pseudo-medical practices. I still wanted to *write* them out of business. Christians, especially, need to be informed because holistic medicine represents itself as being a caring, Christian medical practice, but holistic medicine, as practiced by the American Holistic Medical Association, is neither caring nor Christian. Because holistic medicine is founded in Eastern mysticism and occult practices, it is dangerous and unhealthy for Christians.

For years afterward and still today, every time I hear a news program or see an article in a newspaper or magazine lauding a holistic medical treatment (they always make it sound so appealing), I write, describing my unholy experience with their practices.

In time, an article I wrote exposing the unholy methods carried out by my holistic medical practitioners was published in the *Journal of Christian Nursing*. It detailed the harm I suffered while under their care. Several other magazines, including *SCP Journal* (Spiritual Counterfeits Project), reprinted the article. Later, Greenhaven Press contacted me. They were preparing a health textbook for use in American colleges and universities. They stated that it was hard to find articles opposing alternative care and wanted to reprint my article in their book. I readily consented.

Subsequently, whenever I wrote a letter of rebuttal to a TV station or to a publication advising them to investigate holistic medicine in more depth, I always included a copy of my *Journal of Christian Nursing* article. I have educated a lot of people but have *not* put holistic medicine out of business, as I had hoped to do. Still, I continue to try.

Some people contend that Christians should seek Christian doctors for all their medical needs, but I question that practice. Christians expect their pastors to be Christian, but one's doctor should be well versed in accepted allopathic medical practices. Doctors Jim and Mary, while claiming to be Christian doctors, dabbled in alternative and unorthodox practices outside of Christian beliefs and orthodox medical practices. It took a long time for me to realize they did *not* follow the Hippocratic Oath: "First, do no harm."

Dr. Fields, who guided me through my medical nightmare, was Jewish. Although some of my friends and many of my acquaintances believed I was undergoing a mental breakdown, only Dr. Fields and I felt my condition was neither mental nor emotional but a physical condition that contributed to the other two behaviors. While I didn't have a *mental* breakdown; I will concede I probably had a *nervous* breakdown—that is, all my nerves were breaking down because of the widespread B vitamin imbalance. Only an all-knowing, all-seeing, all-loving God could have directed us to find the key to discovering it.

For a long time, I berated myself, who I considered to be a normally intelligent human being, for being so stupid as to fall for this pseudo-medical philosophy that taught, "*You* can be in control of your life and your health." Then one day, I heard a financial scammer reveal his strategy: "The smartest guys are the easiest targets for a scam," he said, "because they think they are *too smart* to be scammed."

Our downfall, of course, is pride, one of the seven deadly sins. I too thought I was too smart to be fooled, yet I became a victim. Because I wanted to believe that I could be in control of my life and my health, *they sucked me in like quicksand.*

Human nature would have us believe *we* can take control of our lives. Like Adam and Eve in the Garden of Eden, we often listen to Satan, in his different disguises, beguiling us into believing that we can *be* God, instead of merely serving Him. The eternal conflict we struggle with each day: *God's will or my will?*

Had God put me in the wrong place for the right reason and then protected me from death? Joseph's story from the Old Testament often comes to mind: *They meant it for evil, but God meant it for good.*

Someone had to tell the *horrors of holistic medicine.* I decided I would be the one.

Occasionally, I think about the message I received before surgery: "The cancer is not in your ovaries." Where was it then? Was it in my church? Was it in holistic medicine? Was it in my inability to conquer the hate that raged within my soul? I'm still not sure. But the cancer was not in my body—and for that, I will always be grateful.

"I love the Lord, because he has heard my voice and my supplications.

Because he inclined his ear to me, therefore I will call on him as long as I live. The snares of death encompassed me; the pangs of Sheol laid hold on me; I suffered distress and anguish. Then I called on the name of the Lord: 'Lord, I beseech thee, save my life!'"(Psalm 116:1–4 RSV).

"Praise be to God, who has not rejected my prayer or withheld his love from me!" (Psalm 66:20 NIV).

MY LETTER TO THE ARIZONA NURSING ASSOCIATION

This is the letter I wrote to the Arizona Nurses Association, registering my first formal complaint about the care I received at the hands of my nurse practitioner at Arcadia Clinic.

June 16, 1982

Dear Sir or Madam:

I wish to register a formal complaint against Nurse Practitioner Betty Miller, FNP, and against Arcadia Clinic, who is allowing said nurse practitioner to practice medicine without a doctor's license. Both she and the doctors on staff she consults with, if she indeed does consult, are making some serious misdiagnoses. I cite my case as an example.

I began attending Arcadia Clinic in 1965, then known by a different name. Dr. Jim Berry was my physician at the time. In December 1974, I consulted Dr. Jim Berry for abdominal pain. At that time I was given a complete medical exam and diagnosed as having anemia. For treatment, I was advised to take Ferrous Plus, an iron preparation supplied to me by the clinic. After taking this tablet preparation on a daily basis for about a year, I was advised I could discontinue taking it—that I no longer needed it. Later, I learned from CBC reports that my hemoglobin count was 12.0 when I began the treatment and 12.0 when I was told to discontinue the medication. During that year's treatment, the hemoglobin had dropped to a low of 10.8. Was I ever referred to a hematologist for further studies? No.

In June 1976, when I consulted the clinic for my yearly pap smear and in-between period bleeding, I was seen by FNP Betty Miller, who I was told was qualified to perform this type of medical "screening" for the doctors. A polyp of the cervix was found and removed by Betty. From this time until October 23, 1981, Betty Miller or one of the other nurse practitioners on staff over the years treated me as a doctor would. During this time, the only time I remember being seen by a doctor was when Dr. Mary Berry checked the first polyp removed by Betty; later polyp removals were checked by no one. Even when I asked to be seen by Dr. Jim Berry, I was informed that he did not have time to see all his former patients and that the nurse practitioners were duly qualified for this type of office visit. I was lulled into a feeling of trust and security that these were qualified medical people I was consulting; only in this past year did I learn just how unqualified they were, and it could have cost me my life if I had continued to trust them.

Betty wrote numerous prescriptions for me on pads containing Dr. Mary Berry's pre-signed signature. Some of the prescriptions were for Thyrolar, Entozyme, and Ogen (both cream and 2.5 mg tablets)—these are not over-the-counter drugs. When I questioned this practice, I was assured this was within the legal limits of the nurse practitioner's rights, and I did not verify it further.

In May 1980, after losing ten pounds in one month without reason, I consulted Betty Miller at Arcadia Clinic and had a complete blood count (CBC) taken and was pronounced anemic, a condition for which she had treated me off and on for several years, but she never tried to resolve the anemia. At this time, my hemoglobin registered 11.6, well below the 13.5 reading she said I should have. In addition to three (200 mg each) tablets of Vitron C per day, she decided I should also get weekly iron and liver shots. After a month or two, I was feeling decidedly more fatigued, my red cell count had not risen appreciably, and I was experiencing shortness of breath, so Betty decided to add

B12 to my weekly shot. I was also still taking the three Vitron C tablets each day, plus a variety of other vitamins and calcium pills. After one month on the iron, liver, and B12 shots, I was experiencing "fuzziness" (mental dullness) in my head and some eye irregularities (focusing was unclear at times). When I mentioned these complaints to Betty, she reacted by prescribing over-the-counter sinus medication (Triminicin). As I started into the fourth month of shots and tablets, I asked, "How long will I have to continue taking these shots?" She replied, "As long as you need them." My hemoglobin count at this time was 12.5, not even one point higher than when I started. By the fifth month, I was experiencing such mental numbness and inability to concentrate that I was beginning to feel like a walking zombie. I finally got a book from the public library about anemia and learned that iron medication should not be continued longer than *three months* without at least a two-point increase in hemoglobin count. (By this time, mine had slipped back to 11.9—almost what it was when I started the iron regimen.) B12 shots should not be given longer than one month without a dramatic improvement. Betty had prescribed the iron shots for me for *five months* and the B12 shots for *three months* on a weekly basis. I have since learned that with the oral and intravenous iron, some days I was getting ten times the normal therapeutic dosage of iron. I also learned iron should *not* be taken by mouth and injection concurrently. My "doctor" was making me very sick!

I called the Arizona Medical Association and asked for the name of a hematologist. The referral service gave me the name of Dr. Victor Fields. Dr. Fields asked me to bring the results of previous CBCs with me. From my records, I supplied him with Arcadia Clinic dates going back to eight years ago, when Dr. Jim Berry first treated me for anemia. All of the tests indicated that my red cells were normachromic, normacytic—characteristic of hemolytic (cell destruction) anemia, not iron deficiency. I *never* had iron deficiency anemia in the entire eight years of treatment—Dr. Fields confirmed this fact, based on the CBCs provided. Never once in these eight years did anyone at Arcadia Clinic even suggest that I should consult a hematologist, even when I asked, "What is causing this anemia?" Their stock answer was, "Your body doesn't seem to utilize iron properly," and I trusted them enough to accept this explanation.

In the course of his investigation to find the cause of my anemia, Dr. Fields suggested I consult a gynecologist since I had complained of severe abdominal pain during my menses.

For several years, I had consulted Arcadia Clinic for acute abdominal pain and constipation during my menses. Betty suspected endometriosis, but not once did she refer me to a gynecologist. Instead she assured me the endometriosis pain would disappear with the endometriosis if I could "stand the pain" until I finished menopause. (I was just past forty at this time.) She assured me there was "no reason for surgery." Her prescription to alleviate the pain, which she believed was caused by constipation, was Fletcher's Castoria and castor oil packs, applied to the abdominal area with heat (heating pad). The constipation, she said, was caused by the engorgement of the endometrium tissue. She had a plausible explanation for everything, and I didn't know enough not to believe her. I trusted her as the medical authority, foolishly now, I find.

On March 23, I consulted with Dr. John Lance, a gynecologist, who immediately found a large abdominal mass in my left ovary. Because of my anemia, he immediately considered cancer and suggested immediate surgery, after first having ultrasound, liver, and kidney tests performed. The surgery was performed on April 12. He found a grapefruit-size, thin-walled "chocolate" cyst, which burst when they were removing it. If it had burst internally before surgery, he said, it would have created an emergency situation similar to a ruptured appendix. The endometriosis had caused so much infection and inflammation that the entire abdominal cavity was filled with adhesions—they practically had to "skin" the bowel and bladder. The cyst was already deviating the left ureter and the entire pelvic structures were "bound to the pelvic and inferoposterior sidewalls." Because it was bound so securely to the left ureter at this time, a small piece of ovary had to be left attached for fear of damaging the ureter permanently. Even the pelvic bone had to be scraped to eliminate all the endometriosis tissue. The left fallopian tube was completely fused shut, and the right one was in the process of becoming fused shut.

When I consulted Arcadia Clinic in 1974 for abdominal pain, I questioned Dr. Jim Berry whether this pain might be in the ovary because, at the time, my husband and I were trying to get pregnant. Not once did he suggest that endometriosis might be a cause or that it could prevent pregnancy, nor did he suggest further evaluation by a gynecologist.

Approximately two years ago, on June 19 or 20, I consulted Arcadia Clinic for acute abdominal pain and constipation. At that time a rectal exam that was exceedingly painful was performed. Betty's diagnosis was "possible ovarian cyst, possible endometriosis," yet she did not refer me to a gynecologist or in any way indicate that it could be a serious, possibly life-threatening problem.

Dr. Lance told me that without surgery, I soon would have had serious *permanent* kidney and bowel damage. I wonder how much pain and damage from the endometriosis could have been averted if I had been referred to a gynecologist two years sooner; if I had been referred eight years sooner, I might be a mother today.

When I called Betty about the anemia misdiagnosis after my first visit to the hematologist, her flip answer was, "All doctors make mistakes," and when she found I was not in a jovial mood, she said, "Well, you know I didn't make all these decisions by myself. I consulted with Dr. Mary Berry." I have no way of knowing if she consulted with Dr. Mary Berry; she did not do it in my presence, but if she did, as I told her, "That doesn't give me any more confidence in Dr. Mary than it does in you."

Not only are the nurse practitioners on the staff of Arcadia Clinic incompetent to make accurate diagnoses, but the whole clinic staff seems incompetent. Anemia is not a new disease. You'd think even nurses would know how to tell the difference between the three types of anemia (iron deficiency, pernicious, and hemolytic) if they had done their homework. And if they had an anemic patient who was not responding to standard treatment, you would certainly expect them to do a little research or refer the patient. I told Betty she didn't know enough to even know when to refer. It appears that Dr. Jim Berry and Dr. Mary Berry also fall into that category, or they just don't care about patient welfare.

I can't help but wonder how many other Arcadia Clinic patients are being similarly misdiagnosed and mistreated and what long-term effects this will have on their lives.

I have the gynecologist's medical report on my surgery if you would like to have it for your analysis of this complaint, and I will be happy to give you permission to get any information needed from my files with Dr. Fields, Dr. Lance, or Arcadia Clinic. My goal is simply to put Nurse Practitioner Betty Miller out of the "doctoring" business. If you see other medical problems that need correcting, I will be glad to help you pursue this case. Please let me know if there are other formal papers I need to file.

Sincerely,
June B. Schmidt

cc: Arizona Medical Association

MY LETTER TO DR. JOHNSON, NEUROLOGIST

This is the letter I wrote to the neurologist, explaining my thoughts about my B vitamin deficiency theory.

December 28, 1982

Dear Dr. Johnson:

You asked me to write and let you know the results of my B vitamin deficiency theory and the brewer's yeast treatment. So far, it seems to be working.

I returned to the library in hopes of finding the article I thought verified my theory that when the body is overdosed on one B vitamin, it causes the depletion of all B vitamins from the system. Unfortunately, I did not find it—at least not in those words. What I did find was: "Water soluble vitamins—the Bs and Cs—dissolve in water. For the most part, the body simply excretes what it doesn't need in urine and sweat. However, researchers are beginning to find side effects from large doses of water-soluble vitamins, too" (*McCall's*, November 1979), and "Research conducted in the past 15 years indicates that in the U.S. alone, more than 10 million women using oral contraceptives (or female hormones) may need additional amounts of Vitamins B1, B2, C, and folic acid, and as much as two to 10 times the normal amount of vitamin B6" (*Science Digest*, July 1979).

Nutritionist Adelle Davis, in her book *Let's Eat Right to Keep Fit*[16], further states, "The action of all the B vitamins is *synergistic*. One alone or several together increase the need for the B vitamins not supplied (p. 100)...no person is deficient in any one B vitamin without being deficient in all of them ... because these vitamins are needed equally by all cells, a deficiency can produce severe damage before the condition can be noticed. The damage is nevertheless real. Instead of one organ showing abnormalities, as do the eyes, during a vitamin A deficiency, the *entire body degenerates* (emphasis mine) into a one-hoss collapse. This overall abnormality is difficult to recognize in an adult ...(p. 62)"

The question remains, what caused the imbalance? Several possibilities exist. (1) the overdose of unneeded B12 shots administered weekly by my doctor for three months when only one to three *micro*grams are needed daily; (2) the administration of high doses of unneeded estrogen by the same doctor, without the addition of supplemental vitamin B6; (3) an overdose of thyroid medication; or (4) the use of multivitamin and B vitamin supplements, in which the B ratio is not balanced, which also was recommended by my uninformed doctor.

When I reported my symptoms to Dr. John Lance, my gynecologist, he immediately recognized the B6 deficiency and increased my intake to 200 milligrams a day. Prior to that, I was taking 100 milligrams—50 milligrams in the morning and 50 milligrams in the evening. He had added B6 to my treatment after I returned home, just after the first major bout with vertigo in Wisconsin. I had noticed the immediate calming effect soon after starting the B6 treatment, like a tranquilizer. The second bout of vertigo happened in November, but thinking back, I realized that I had been forgetting to take the afternoon B6 dosage. In effect, I was reducing my B6 intake to 50 milligrams a day. Adelle Davis says B6 is needed to convert the amino acid, tryptophan, to niacin. Niacin, or nicotinic acid, is often used in the treatment of vertigo problems.

---

[16] Adelle Davis, AB, MS. *Let's Eat Right to Keep Fit* (New York: Harcourt, Brace and Company, 1954).

My B deficiency, I believe, is more than just B6, however, because even taking the increased dosage of B6, I still experienced abdominal discomfort—constipation, gas, flatulence—and continued occasional mental "fuzziness" or dullness. You will remember that I stated that the dizziness and nausea seemed somewhat relieved by bowel movement/s. Until I learned of the B vitamin deficiency, I could not see the correlation of this syndrome. Even stool softeners and mild laxative did not always seem helpful with my bowel problems, and I was opposed to being forced to rely on these artificial aids anyway.

Adelle Davis explains: "A deficiency of B1 causes digestive disturbances in a number of ways. Energy production is so faulty that muscular contractions of the stomach and intestinal walls slow down; food can no longer be well mixed with digestive juices and enzymes; and the already digested food cannot be brought into frequent contact with the absorbing surface where it can pass into the blood...interference with energy production so limits the contractions of the walls of the large intestine that waste material remains in the large bowel longer than it should ... the harder and drier the stools become ...constipation."[17]

She further explains on page 62: "The reason for personality changes and such symptoms as mental depression, confused thinking, and forgetfulness which occur when vitamin B is undersupplied is twofold: first, brain cells derive their energy only from sugar, and glucose cannot be converted into energy without this vitamin [the reason, possibly, for my hypoglycemic reactions in October 1981]; second, the accumulation of pyruvic and lactic acids in the brain cells is somewhat *toxic*." (Emphasis is mine—the reason for my mental "fuzziness" and inability to focus.)

With a cholin deficiency, hemorrhages are produced, which may explain the blood accumulation under my big toenails in October 1981.

Just before Thanksgiving, I began taking two teaspoons of brewer's yeast in the morning in a glass of "tiger's milk" (juice glass of milk; juice

---

[17] Ibid, 104-105

glass of orange juice, half a banana—blended). Within five days my bowel movements had improved to the point where I was able to give up all stool softeners. On days when the afternoon "fuzzies" recurred, I also took a teaspoon or two of brewer's yeast in a glass of orange juice. Within an hour, the "fuzzies" disappeared.

For quite a while, I also supplemented my diet with a half cup of yogurt at noon. Adelle Davis recommends this for people with severe digestive disturbances, and because I had suffered with constipation for many years, I figured mine was severe. Also, I was having some problems with canker sores, and from past experience, I knew they healed more rapidly when I ate yogurt. (According to Adelle Davis, canker sores are caused by a niacin deficiency—why don't doctors know that? Yogurt contains the essential B vitamins and digestive aids to release niacin into the system. When I was first diagnosed anemic eight years ago, I had consulted my holistic doctor because of severe canker and mouth sores.)

When I discussed the possibility of a B vitamin deficiency with Dr. Fields, he at first rejected the B12 overdose as a possibility but later agreed that a thyroid overdose could cause it. Since we had reduced my thyroid dosage at the October 15 visit, another thyroid test was conducted December 17. The T4 reading had dropped from 6.4 to 5.4 and although this was still within the low normal range, he doesn't feel thyroid overdose is responsible. However, since reducing the thyroid dosage, my body doesn't feel like I am running in "high gear" all the time anymore. Remember, I noted that after reducing the thyroid dosage, I reverted from my "usual" insomniac self to sleeping so soundly I felt almost drugged.

I have now been on brewer's yeast for more than a month. I have increased the dosage to one heaping tablespoon a day, which I take in the morning (with tiger's milk) when I first get up. My body tissues seem to have absorbed the excess B vitamins now and I seldom need an "afternoon feeding," except the B6 which is taken with supper.

I have noticed a number of improvements in my general well-being:

less body itching (eczema); tongue coating is gradually disappearing, as are tongue crevices; improved concentration and organization; fewer feelings of panic if all my projects don't get finished in a day; no vertigo; no nausea; no vomiting; depression and mood swings diminished; forgetfulness still needs improvement though canker and mouth sores healed; energy levels are building; headaches reduced; bone pains improved; chapped lips improved; less gas and flatulence; softer stools. (My stools usually move within thirty minutes after taking the brewer's yeast each day. When I was taking the afternoon dosage, they moved again then and sometimes between those two dosages. Adelle Davis notes that this increased activity indicates a severe deficiency.)

B vitamin deficiencies can also produce anemia and an elevated sedimentation rate, caused by the putrefactive intestinal bacteria. In mid-January, I am due for my regular three-month blood test. It will be interesting to see if there is an improvement in either or both tests.

Where do you suggest I submit my paper?

As a matter of fact, I am writing a book about my experiences and my findings, which I hope will be an eye-opener to the general public.

Thank you for your part in my treatment, though I hope you understand if I say I hope I never have to see you again, at least as a patient. It was necessary for me to know the tests you performed were normal before concentrating on the B vitamin deficiency theory. I suppose there is no way to know for sure if permanent nerve or other damage has resulted from this deficiency until new symptoms appear. I plan to continue with the daily brewer's yeast—possibly for the rest of my life. It is a small price to pay for good health.

Very truly yours,
June B. Schmidt

cc: Dr. V. Fields
Dr. J. Lance

Note: I never had to return to Dr. Johnson.